ESSENTIAL OILS
-*for*-
HORMONE BLISS

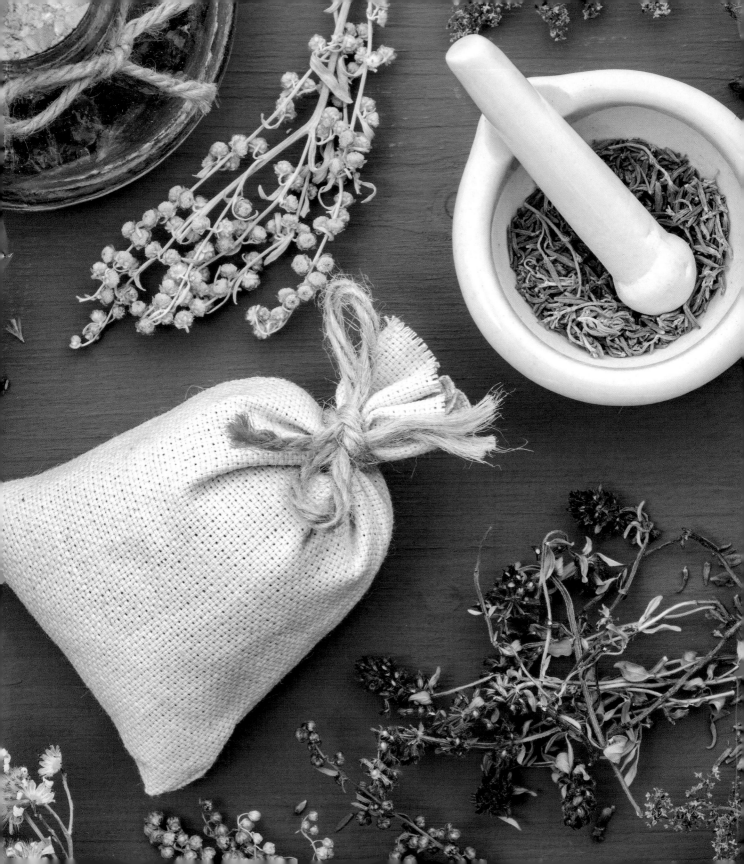

ESSENTIAL OILS

-for-

HORMONE BLISS

Boost Your Energy,
Lose Weight Naturally,
and Improve Your Sleep

Michelle Schoffro Cook, PhD, DNM

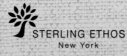

STERLING ETHOS
New York

DEDICATION

To my sister, Bobbi-Jo Meyer

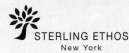

STERLING ETHOS
New York

An Imprint of Sterling Publishing Co., Inc.
122 Fifth Avenue
New York. NY 10011

ISBN 978-1-4549-3825-5
978-1-4549-3826-2 (e-book)

Distributed in Canada by Sterling Publishing Co., Inc.
C/o Canadian Manda Group, 664 Annette Street
Toronto, Ontario M6S 2C8, Canada
Distributed in the United Kingdom by GMC Distribution Services
Castle Place, 166 High Street, Lewes, East Sussex BN7 1XU, England
Distributed in Australia by NewSouth Books
University of New South Wales, Sydney, NSW 2052, Australia

For information about custom editions, special sales, and premium
and corporate purchases, please contact Sterling Special Sales
at 800-805-5489 or specialsales@sterlingpublishing.com.

Manufactured in Spain

2 4 6 8 10 9 7 5 3 1

sterlingpublishing.com

Cover design by Elizabeth Mihaltse Lindy

Interior design by Christine Heun

Picture credits on page 177

CONTENTS

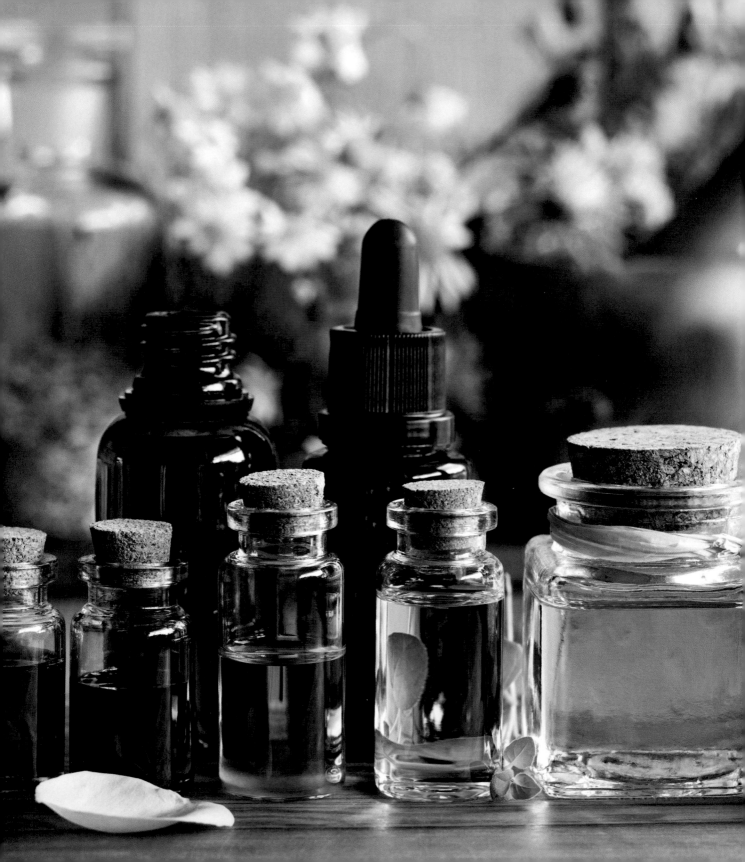

Introduction

From Hormone Hell
to Hormone Well

DO YOU FEEL LIKE AN EMOTIONAL WRECK EVEN WHEN nothing apparent is going wrong? Do you frequently feel as though you can't cope with life's stresses or feel overwhelmed with your responsibilities? Do you suffer from painful or irregular periods, or mood swings? Perhaps you experience hot flashes and an inability to sleep, along with brain fog and memory lapses. Or perhaps you find it hard to lose weight no matter what diet you try or how much you exercise. If you're suffering from any of these symptoms, then you may be experiencing the effects of a hormonal imbalance. It's not all in your head.

What if you could naturally and effectively balance your hormones for good—no more weight gain, hair falling out, cold hands and feet, depression, mood swings, PMS, menopausal symptoms, low libido, a low sense of attractiveness, or difficulty getting a good night's sleep? Well, you can finally start experiencing the quality of life you were born to live thanks to the information contained in this book.

Whether you're suffering from hypothyroidism, hyperthyroidism, adrenal fatigue, menopausal symptoms, PMS, andropause, blood sugar imbalances, and many other hormonal-related health issues, you'll find the relief you seek in *Essential Oils for Hormone Bliss*. Essential oils can offer a powerful way to address the hormonal imbalances behind your symptoms. When used correctly, they work quickly and effectively, and are free from the lengthy lists of side effects linked to pharmaceutical drugs.

Essential oils can have many effects in the body: they can affect brain hormones that affect the glands, reduce the effects of stress and the stress hormones secreted by the adrenal glands, support the healthy and balanced functioning of the glands in the body, and even stimulate the glands to secrete more of the hormones they need for your body to function optimally.

Though it may seem implausible, essential oils are, arguably, some of the most powerful natural medicines on the planet, particularly when the best and purest oils are used, in the ideal application to obtain the desired results, and in the correct dose. I started using essential oils in my holistic nutrition and natural medicine practice just over two decades ago. I have worked with thousands of clients over the years. I refer to these people as "clients" rather than "patients" as most doctors do because I believe in the power of words. I want them to recognize that they have a tremendous amount of power over their healing, understand that I am someone who will help them along their journey, and attempt to eliminate any perceived hierarchy that is common in the doctor–patient relationship.

Twenty years ago alternative medicine was not the popular thing it is now. Conversely, it was a last resort for most people who had tried everything that Western pharmaceutical medicine had to offer and were still suffering from health issues. To say that I received the "tough" cases would be

an understatement, but I didn't mind at all. I saw helping these people as a challenge. More importantly, it was an opportunity to help those who had been largely neglected or forgotten by the medical community, ignored or abandoned by the people to whom they turned for help.

Due to their disillusionment with the medical system, many of these people were open to using nutrition, lifestyle changes, and natural medicines to address their suffering. I counselled them in these modalities, helping them to discover the inherent healing ability of their body when it is treated in a way that is harmonious with nature.

As a result of working with so many diverse people, I have had the joy of witnessing many huge health transformations using essential oils. While dietary and lifestyle changes alone often had impressive outcomes, I observed astounding results when I incorporated essential oils into their regimens. This was almost unheard of at the time and even now is sometimes the target of unwarranted criticism or controversy. Women whose hot flashes didn't respond to medication or herbs experienced rapid relief using essential oils. People whose adrenal fatigue was so severe that they could barely function experienced significant improvement in their energy levels. Those who suffered from insomnia that interfered with their ability to perform their work tasks the following days experienced deep and restorative sleep. These are just a few of the improvements I witnessed in my practice. Even though I was aware of how powerful essential oils can be, their success

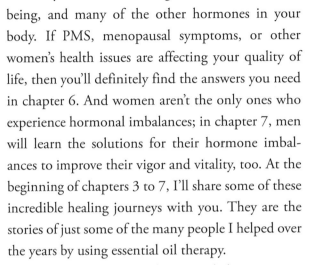

stories continued to surprise and amaze me. I receive regular e-mails and messages from people around the world who write to tell me how the essential oils I have recommended in my practice and through my writing have transformed their health and lives.

In the coming chapters, I'll share my knowledge about essential oils gathered from more than twenty-five years' experience in medical aromatherapy—a scientific approach to aromatherapy that employs the healing power of natural chemical constituents found in key essential oils and includes the topical use, diffusing, and ingestion of appropriate oils to get optimal results. Corporations in the bath and beauty industry have led most people to believe that aromatherapy is beneficial for relaxation, skin care, and bathing. While it can definitely be used for these purposes, medical aromatherapy can dramatically affect the health of the glands, our stress levels and our ability to cope with stress, our capacity to get deep and restorative sleep, our body's natural ability to restore our natural hormonal balance, and even brain health.

In chapter 1, you'll discover the healing power of essential oils and how to start benefiting from them immediately. Next, in chapter 2, you'll discover my 10-Day Plan for Hormone Perfection, which will help you to lay the foundation for great hormonal health. In chapter 3, you'll learn how to rejuvenate your body's stress glands—the adrenals—for more energy and a better ability to cope with stress and its myriad effects. If you've ever suspected that your weight gain, thinning hair, and feeling cold might be linked to a hormonal imbalance, you'll find everything you need to reset your thyroid gland in chapter 4. In chapter 5, you'll learn about the brain hormones that control your moods, feelings of well-being, and many of the other hormones in your body. If PMS, menopausal symptoms, or other women's health issues are affecting your quality of life, then you'll definitely find the answers you need in chapter 6. And women aren't the only ones who experience hormonal imbalances; in chapter 7, men will learn the solutions for their hormone imbalances to improve their vigor and vitality, too. At the beginning of chapters 3 to 7, I'll share some of these incredible healing journeys with you. They are the stories of just some of the many people I helped over the years by using essential oil therapy.

While it may seem a bit overwhelming to get started, I will walk you through everything you need to know to achieve hormonal balance and experience an amazing quality of life with essential oils. It gives me great pleasure to introduce the hormonal healing power of essential oils to you and to help you regain the quality of life you deserve. Not only are you likely to feel much better, you'll also love the sensual journey to great health when you follow the recipes found in the boxes throughout this book.

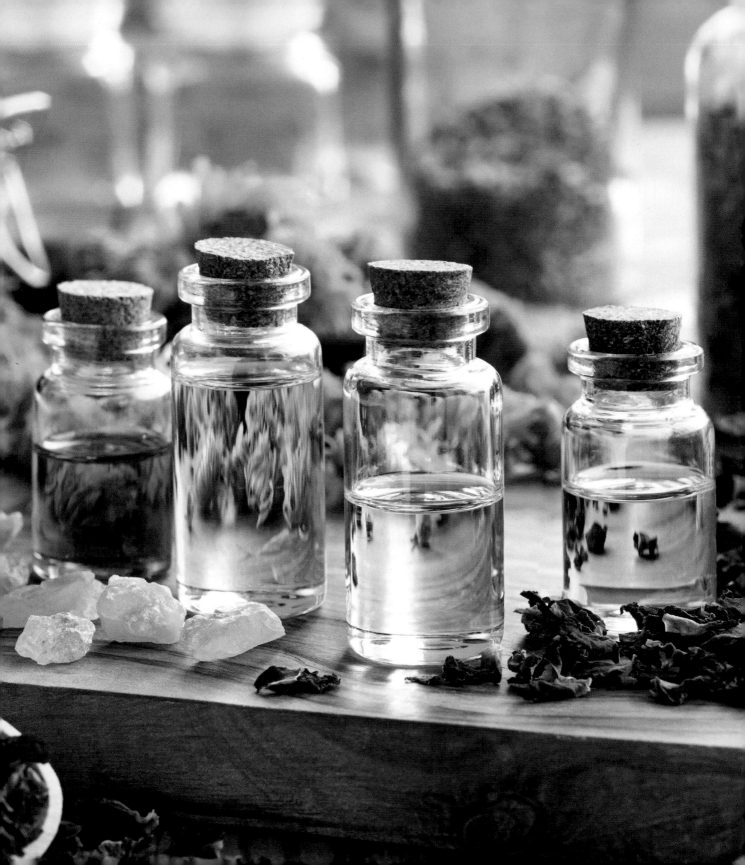

Essential Oils 101

An Overview of the Basics

Some people have the misguided notion that they need to have a complete course of study in essential oils to benefit from their use. That belief could not be further from the truth. That said, it does help to have an overview of essential oils and their healing abilities. Let's get started.

A Brief History of Aromatherapy and Essential Oils

Aromatherapy is the therapeutic use of natural oils from flowers, plants, trees, resins, and other botanical elements in nature that have healing properties. These are known as essential oils.

Essential oils have unique therapeutic traits. Different essential oils can contain hundreds of chemical constituents, each of which produces unique effects in the body. Even the same plant grown in different conditions can result in different chemical constituents and therefore different therapeutic effects. Each plant can also produce more than one type of oil, depending on the parts used in the oil extraction process: for example, the leaves may yield different healing properties than an oil extracted from the flowers on the same plant. But it isn't necessary to understand the complex chemistry of the plants and their oils to reap the healing rewards they offer.

Humans have been using the art and science of aromatherapy therapeutically for at least 6,000 years. There is plenty of archaeological evidence to suggest that aromatherapy oils were regularly used in the ancient temples of Egypt, Greece, and Rome. Our ancient ancestors must have observed that the scents of flowers, trees, and other plants had an impact on their stress levels, anxiety, sleep, mood, pain, and more.

Not only is aromatherapy one of the most powerful and fast-acting medical therapies available due to the thousands of active compounds as well as their timely absorption through the skin or through inhalation, it can be a supremely enjoyable experience.

Naturally fragrant essential oils absorb through the skin into the bloodstream during massage. Alternatively, they can be diffused into the air where they are inhaled through our nose, giving many of the molecules direct and quick access to the brain. Thanks to our drug-, surgery-, and radiation-based system of medicine, most of us have been led to believe that medicine must be harsh to be effective; aromatherapy seems too pleasurable to be effective medicine but because it quickly gains access to the blood and brain, impressive results are commonplace and fast-acting. And, if we choose pure oils suitable for internal use, they can be used, not just safely, but most effectively to achieve astounding health results.

Over the last several decades, research at some of the world's leading universities has found that essential oils are effective for pain, inflammation, infection, depression, dementia, and many other symptoms and conditions we experience.

Three Categories of Essential Oils

Oils are frequently divided into three main classifications depending on their properties.

Uplifting Oils

Uplifting oils boost mood and energy levels and are often helpful for the symptoms of depression or low energy that often accompany hormonal imbalances. These oils can give our glands the boost they sometimes need to work more effectively. That's where these oils can be helpful. If you are suffering from these symptoms, or just a general lack of motivation, then you'll probably want to explore some of these oils. Peppermint and most of the citrus oils, including bergamot, grapefruit, lemon, neroli, and wild orange, fall into this category.

Balancing Oils

Balancing oils tend to regulate hormones and brain messengers known as neurotransmitters. You'll learn more about these powerful hormone-regulating oils throughout this book. If you know you're suffering from hormonal imbalances, aren't sure where to begin, feel overwhelmed, and just need some emotional and physical balancing, you'll find that balancing oils offer tremendous support. Some balancing oils include frankincense and clary sage.

Calming Oils

Calming oils tend to relax the nervous system. Some even have sedative properties that can improve sleep quality. Some examples of calming oils include lavender and vetiver. These oils can be helpful in the treatment of chronic stress, anxiety, sleep disorders, and insomnia.

Many oils span multiple categories and can have any combination of uplifting, balancing, and calming properties. For example, while frankincense has balancing properties, many people find that it is calming as well. You may also discover that you benefit from using different types of the essential oils. That is fine too. While many people are often intimidated by the prospect of using essential oils, the reality is that they tend to be quite safe and there are rarely ever any negative side effects, particularly when only the highest quality oils are used.

Choosing High-Quality Oils

It is important to choose high-quality essential oils, as lower-quality, inexpensive oils have greatly diminished therapeutic effects. While there are many types of oils in the marketplace, few are produced to maintain the integrity of the plant. Many essential oils are contaminated with solvents used during extraction, plant matter from the incorrect species of an herb, and toxic chemicals like hormone-disrupting and cancer-causing phthalates. Some may have also been diluted with cheap, unwanted oils that are not suitable for ingestion.

Avoid oils from some large bath and body product shops. They tend to be extremely low grade, are frequently diluted with cheaper oils, and often contain synthetic or toxic ingredients, which can throw off hormones even further, worsen existing health conditions, or cause additional unwanted health concerns. You won't find these toxic ingredients listed on the label so it's hard to know if you're buying a quality product.

You'll also want to avoid products that are labeled "fragrance" oils, "perfume" oils, or "natural identical" oils. They are usually made from synthetic chemicals that offer no therapeutic value whatsoever. Likewise, many cheap options contain synthetic versions of the oils, which also offer no therapeutic value and may actually be harmful. Worse than that, many cheap oils, especially those from department stores, pharmacies, and bath and beauty shops, are adulterated with petrochemical solvents used during the extraction process or toxic pesticides used to grow the herbs from which the oils are extracted.

When it comes to essential oils, you get what you pay for. If you buy something cheap, you probably aren't getting a product that will help restore balance to your hormones; it may even exacerbate your hormonal health problems or contain carcinogens.

Many unscrupulous companies even inaccurately list ingredients or plant species. For example, you could be thinking you're buying melissa essential oil when you're actually getting lemongrass, which has few of the same health effects or benefits. Or, the birch essential oil in your shopping cart may actually be wintergreen essential oil, which is much cheaper.

Where can you find undiluted, pure essential oils? Look for a company that insists on several methods of independent third-party testing to ensure the purity, integrity, and potency of their oils, and that the oils are unadulterated. The essential oil market is a bit of a wild west when it comes to the large number of untrustworthy companies and potentially adulterated products. Avoid the essential oil products in most department stores, pharmacies, and bath and beauty shops. Buy from a company that specializes in essential oils and oil-related products and provides customers with extensive educational materials, customer support, and third-party testing of their products. However, keep in mind that some companies claim their products are "pure" or "natural," but that these terms mean nothing as there are no regulatory quality control standards that companies need to meet to make these claims.

Of course, as with anything, you shouldn't use oils that have expired beyond their best-before date as they lose potency over time and may have gone rancid. Choose a product that specifies the correct species of plant on the label, keeping in mind that you'll want to conduct some research to see if third-party laboratory tests confirm that you're actually getting what the label says.

Be sure that the oils you select are also sustainably harvested to ensure that no environmental harm occurs in the harvesting or production of the essential oils. While it is good to choose organic, the reality is that the term "organic" means different things in different countries where the herbs, flowers, or trees are grown, so it may not mean anything.

To ensure the potency, purity, and safety of your essential oils, store them in a dark place away from air, heat, and light, and of course, keep them away from children.

How to Use Essential Oils

Essential oils are highly concentrated and powerful natural medicines. By some estimates, they are between forty and sixty times stronger than the herbs from which they are derived. A little goes a long way so you'll only need a drop or a few at a time, based on the oil and the recipes I've provided.

When using essential oils, it is imperative to follow some basic safety guidelines. It is best to use them as directed on the product label or within this book.

* Always read labels prior to use, and store essential oils away from children and pets.

* Always dilute strong oils like cassia, cinnamon, cloves, geranium, lemongrass, oregano, and thyme, among others, by using a carrier oil such as fractionated coconut oil or apricot kernel oil. A carrier oil is a gentle oil used to dilute essential oils to make them suitable for topical use.

* If you're planning to use them internally, choose only products that indicate their suitability for internal use on the label.

* Avoid applying essential oils in direct contact with the delicate mucous membranes of the eyes and mouth. It's always best to dilute an essential oil and conduct a test by applying a patch on the inner wrist and waiting 48 hours to see if you experience an adverse reaction.

* When used topically, some oils can cause photosensitivity—that means that they can make your skin more sensitive to the sun. These oils typically include citrus oils. Avoid using these oils on your skin within several hours of direct sun exposure.

* If you are pregnant or lactating, you should only use oils that can be safely used during these times. (For general guidelines about using oils during pregnancy or lactation, please see page 9.)

* Always inform your physician and obtain his or her approval for using any oils prior to starting a regimen to ensure they are suitable for you, particularly if you have any health conditions, are pregnant, or breastfeeding.

* Don't discontinue any prescription medications without first consulting your doctor. And, remember that essential oils, while highly effective, should not replace any drugs you're taking.

* The information, recipes, and dosage guidelines contained throughout this book are intended for adults only. Do not use with babies or children without consulting a qualified health practitioner versed in essential oil therapy.

There are three main ways to use essential oils: aromatically (inhaling their lovely scents), topically (on your skin), or internally (either on your tongue, in food or beverages, or in empty capsules). Not all oils are suitable for all types of uses so be sure to read the labels on the products you select.

Aromatic Uses

When you smell essential oils, you're actually breathing in potent oil-based plant extracts of essential oils wafting in the air. They send signals directly from the cells in the nose to the brain. The brain then sends messages back to the body in response to the signals it received. The signals will vary depending on the scent (or scents) and the chemical constituents they contain, and will produce different effects, whether that be reducing inflammation, relaxing the nervous system, enhancing mood, increasing energy, or reducing pain, or some other action depending on the initial chemical constituents detected in the essential oil. Inhaling essential oils is a quick way for their molecules to access the brain—usually in a minute or less—where they can help to quickly restore hormone balance.

The most common way to use essential oils aromatically is to diffuse one to five drops in an oil diffuser. I don't recommend using oil burners as the heat can damage the chemical makeup of the oils, reducing their effectiveness and even causing them to smoke, contributing to health problems as a result. Here are some additional suggestions:

* Mix a 500-milliliter spray bottle of water with eight to ten drops of essential oils, shake thoroughly, and spray on carpets, furniture, and linens. You can also spray your clothing although you'll want to be sure that you shake the mixture well before doing so to avoid staining.

* Place a drop of essential oil on a cotton ball, and place the cotton ball in closets, drawers, or on windowsills to keep unwanted pests like moths away.

* Add a drop or two of your favorite essential oil to an old facecloth (use one that you're not concerned about staining). Place the cloth in the dryer along with your clothes to give a lovely, natural scent to your clothing without the toxic chemicals of fabric softeners. Learn more about the problems of fabric softeners on page 34.

* Add a few drops of eucalyptus or other essential oil around the edges of your shower (not somewhere they'll cause you to slip) for a quick and easy steam inhalation to start your day.

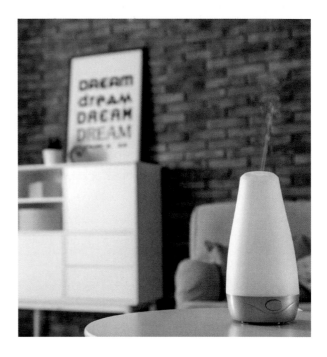

Topical Uses

Applying essential oils on the skin allows them to address local skin conditions but also to quickly penetrate it and gain access to the bloodstream. Here are some of the ways in which you can use essential oils topically:

* Add a drop of your favorite essential oil to a dollop of unscented, toxin-free moisturizer. You can also dilute a drop or two in a carrier oil like fractionated coconut oil. The level of dilution will depend on the oil, the skin sensitivity of the person on which it will be applied, and whether the mixture will be used on a child or adult. One to two drops of essential oil per teaspoon of carrier oil is common and can be applied to skin as a moisturizer, therapeutic treatment, or massage oil. Apply the diluted oils or moisturizer with a drop of essential oil to your abdomen, arms, chest, forehead, legs, temples, and neck; avoid the skin around the eyes (unless you're using a product specifically formulated for this purpose), inner ears, eyes, or broken or damaged skin.

* Put a drop of an essential oil on the palm of your hands or the soles of your feet. This is a convenient way to use the oils and still benefit from their therapeutic and lovely aromas throughout the day.

* Add a few drops of essential oils to a teaspoon of carrier oil and add to a hot bath and soak for ten to twenty minutes.

* Add a couple of drops to an old facecloth that has been soaked in either hot or cold water and wrung out. Use as a hot or cold compress. Cover the compress with a dry cloth to help retain its temperature.

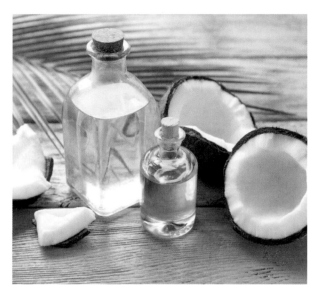

Internal Uses

Most North American essential oil practitioners lack an adequate understanding of essential oils as natural medicines, which often means that they discourage people from using one of the most effective means of using essential oils for hormone transformation—ingestion of suitable oils. I've used these methods in my practice for many years to help women and men put a stop to their seemingly endless and horrible hot flashes, insomnia, depression, and other hormone-related health conditions when nothing else worked. While there are some oils that are not suitable for this purpose and safety precautions to consider, most people ingest some amount of essential oil in the plant-based foods and herbs they eat every day. Plus, essential oils themselves have been used internally throughout history.

When correctly used, ingesting essential oils can

be the most effective way to experience their benefits. Once you ingest a suitable essential oil, the oil compounds enter the bloodstream through the gastrointestinal tract, where they are transported to all the organs and glands, including the brain. I've used ingestible essential oils in my practice for many years, with exceptional results.

As with anything that is consumed, it is imperative to use appropriate doses to avoid toxicity—the point at which even the healthiest of substances becomes unhealthy or harmful. If you're considering using essential oils internally, you'll need to consider whether the one you're using is suitable for internal use, and, if so, how much to use and in which format, whether it is a capsule or a drop of oil taken directly or under the tongue, or another method.

Finding the highest quality essential oils is even more important when you'll be using them internally. Essential oils that are suitable for this purpose will indicate this on the label. If the products you've selected are actually appropriate for internal use, it will have "for internal use," "dosage amount," or something similar on the label. If the label does not indicate anything like that, avoid using them internally since they are likely to have contaminants that are too toxic for such use.

Once you've selected the purest oils, you'll still want to check to be sure the individual oil is suitable for internal use. For example, some brands of high-quality peppermint are fine for internal use, but clary sage should not be used this way. I've included

descriptions and information throughout this book to help you safely and effectively use essential oils. In the meantime, here are some ways to use essential oils internally:

* Essential oils that are extracted from culinary herbs, such as basil, cilantro, peppermint, or rosemary, can be used in place of their herbal counterparts. You'll only need a drop or two in your favorite foods since the oils are potent.

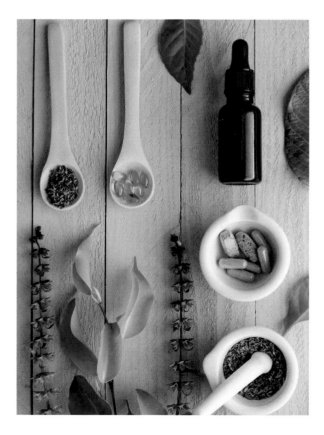

* Add a drop of essential oil of lemon, grapefruit, or your preferred oil to your water and stir it thoroughly for a flavor boost that also ramps up the healing properties of the water you're drinking.

* Place a few drops of essential oils in empty capsules, available in most health food stores. Take the capsules with a glass of water, along with some food. Some oils like cassia, cinnamon, clove, oregano, and thyme all need to be diluted with a little fractionated coconut or olive oil before ingesting. Follow the package label for the specific oil you've selected.

* You can also purchase preformed essential oil supplements to aid digestion, target pain, address sleep issues, or other purposes. Again, it is imperative to exclusively choose products that are high quality for this purpose.

Regardless of why you're using essential oils internally, start slowly using only a drop or two at a time a few times daily. Do not exceed twenty drops in a twenty-four hour period.

Using Essential Oils During Pregnancy and Breastfeeding

You can safely use essential oils during any phase of life, including pregnancy, provided you follow some simple safety precautions. For ethical reasons, there are few studies exploring the safe use of essential oils during these phases of life.

Some women can experience sensitivity to oils during pregnancy that they handled without issues prior to becoming pregnant. It is worth considering if you suspect any increased sensitivity to the oils during pregnancy. You may still be able to use them but may just need to modify how you do so. For example, instead of ingesting the oils, you may be better off diffusing them instead.

If you are unsure about essential oils for use during these times, it is best to work with a qualified natural health professional skilled in the therapeutic use of essential oils.

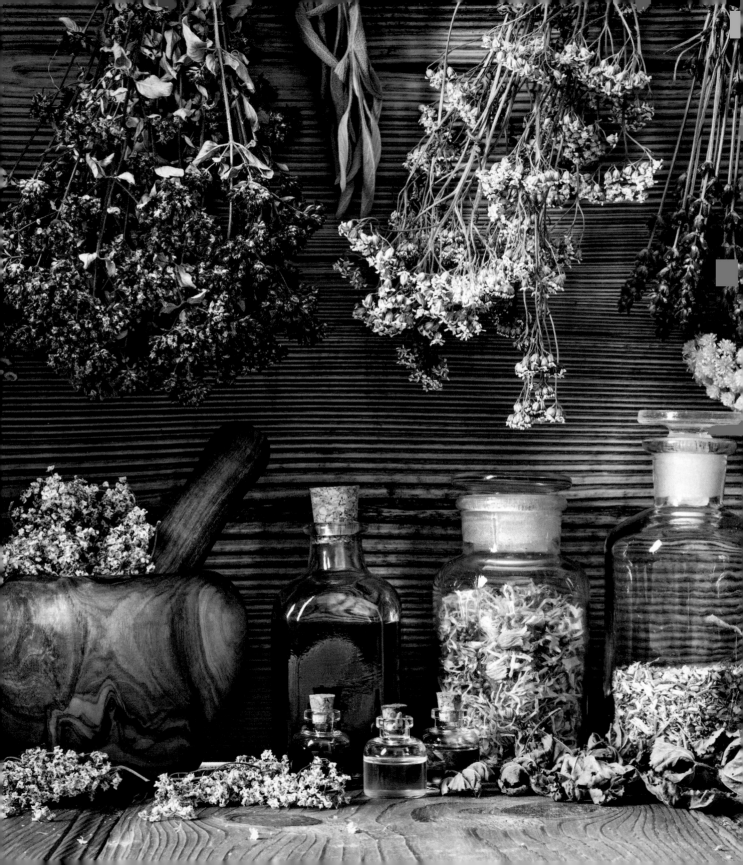

2

What's Going on with Me?

Dr. Cook's 10-Day Plan for Hormone Perfection

BEFORE WE DELVE INTO THE VARIOUS ADRENAL, thyroid, or other hormonal imbalances that may be plaguing you, let's first explore some of the critical factors underlying most hormonal imbalances and how to begin addressing them. In my many years of clinical experience as a doctor of natural medicine and a clinical nutritionist, I have identified four main problems that frequently underlie almost all hormone-related conditions: inflammation, an overburdened liver, blood sugar imbalances, and hormone-disrupting toxin exposures.

Addressing these issues builds the foundation for great health. Of course, there are others, and you will learn more about them in the following chapters of this book, but for now let's start here.

Hormones-at-a-Glance

Hormones are substances that are produced in your body and control the activities of cells, glands, or organs. Essentially, they are chemical messengers in the body. They are produced by glands in the brain known as the pineal gland, pituitary gland, and hypothalamus; adrenal glands (two triangular-shaped glands that sit atop the kidneys); thyroid gland (a butterfly-shaped gland in your neck); and ovaries or testes, among others. Combined, these glands and the hormones they secrete constitute the endocrine system. When they are working smoothly and your hormones are balanced, you feel energetic, sleep deeply at night, awaken refreshed and rejuvenated, regulate body temperature, enjoy a healthy sex drive, and balance your weight. In other words, you feel great.

But, our modern lifestyles, with their chronic stresses and pressures, the chemicals in our food—which already bears little resemblance to what our ancestors ate—can throw off our delicate hormonal balance. Our sedentary lifestyles, poor air quality, and exposure to toxic substances can wreak havoc on our hormones as well. Let's explore some of the common factors that contribute to our imbalanced hormones.

Quell Inflammation at the Source

Everywhere you turn, inflammation is cited as the cause of a serious health condition or a factor that needs to be addressed to maintain good health and to balance hormones, regardless of whether it originates in the brain, adrenal glands, thyroid, or another place in the body.

What Is Inflammation?

Inflammation is the body's means of self-protection, whether from harmful microbes like bacteria, fungi, or viruses; toxins in our food, water, air, pharmaceutical drugs, or street drugs; or free radicals and the damaged cells they cause. Free radicals are unstable molecules that damage surrounding cells and tissue, leading to illness, disease, and premature aging. No matter the cause, the body's immune system uses inflammation to minimize the damage by killing microbes, removing toxins or damaged cells, or neutralizing the free radicals before they can cause further damage.

While inflammation seems to damage the body and is linked to many health conditions, including hormonal imbalances, we need inflammation to survive. Without the inflammatory process, our bodies would not heal from wounds, infections, or other injuries or illness. However, inflammation can become a problem when the immune system cannot control it, the damaged cells and tissues in the body are unable to recover from it, or it occurs over long periods of time.

Signs of Inflammation

When inflammation is the result of external wounds or conditions like arthritis, it is usually characterized by pain, redness, immobility, swelling, and heat. However, not all of these signs may be detectable when the inflammation occurs deep within the body, such as within the gut or the glands, or in the case of hormonal imbalances.

While short-term inflammation may be helpful in addressing the problem that initiated it, chronic inflammation can become a threat to health. Chronic inflammation is a root cause of many diseases and linked to a wide range of hormonal issues like hypothyroidism, adrenal fatigue, menopausal symptoms, and many others, which we'll discuss in the following chapters.

Inflammation is a critical response by the immune system to address injury, fight bacteria or viruses, and heal damaged tissue. The immune system causes blood vessels to dilate, while also bringing white blood cells to the areas of concern so the body can heal the infection, injury, or damage. When inflammation becomes chronic, the immune system can start attacking healthy glands, causing them to lose functionality or to function incorrectly. Additionally, the blood vessels that would otherwise supply healthy glands with oxygen-rich blood and nutrients can narrow with plaque buildup, which can cause the glands to lack the nutrients and oxygen they need to function properly or to manufacture sufficient hormones.

The Link between Your Gut and Inflammation

Your gut plays a critical role in the health of your brain, glands, and hormones—all of which determines the health of your whole body. Beneficial bacteria in your intestines aid digestion, ensure the proper absorption of essential nutrients, eliminate waste products from the intestines, aid the manufacture of critical vitamins, control harmful bacteria and other microbe populations in the body, metabolize excess cholesterol, and quell inflammation. These beneficial bacteria also secrete anti inflammatory compounds that affect the walls of the intestines, which helps to regulate the immune system and prevent overactive responses that lead it to attack the body's own tissues (as is the case with autoimmune disorders like the thyroid condition known as Hashimoto's disease).

When there are insufficient beneficial bacteria in the intestines, harmful bacteria or yeasts may become overgrown, resulting in intestinal infections. The byproducts these microorganisms secrete can damage the walls of the intestines and subject the body to additional inflammation, which can harm the glands or even impact the controller of the glands—the brain. Some of these byproducts even act like hormones, throwing off the hormonal balance in the body. Others create inflammation that, as you learned earlier, can result in the narrowing of blood vessels to the glands, causing them to have a shortage of nutrients that are needed to manufacture hormones. In some cases, the inflammation can cause the immune system to attack the glands.

Gut health is integrally linked to inflammation. A massive body of research shows that it is frequently the result of an imbalance between harmful microbes and beneficial probiotic microbes in the intestines. When this happens, you may be experiencing silent inflammation without even realizing it. Silent inflammation is the type of inflammation that lacks any outward symptoms. Most of the inflammation in our bodies is silent inflammation that we don't even know it is occurring beneath the surface.

Signs You May Have a Gut Bacterial Imbalance

There are many signs that you might have a gut bacterial imbalance. Some of the most common ones include constipation, diarrhea, nausea, upset stomach, indigestion, or sugar cravings. You might be surprised to learn that even conditions such as anxiety, rheumatoid arthritis, lupus, Hashimoto's thyroiditis, fibromyalgia, and irritable bowel syndrome can be linked to a gut bacterial imbalance. Those who suffer from chronic gut bacterial imbalances tend to have a wide variety of symptoms that may be impacting their quality of life.

Science has even started to discover that some of the foods that don't seem to agree with us actually throw off our bacterial balance, which could explain, at least in part, why these foods make us feel bad after eating them. Excess meat, dairy, and sugars are just a few of the types of foods that have this effect. There are many other signs and conditions that indicate your intestines may have an overgrowth of harmful bacteria or yeasts, including:

* Abdominal pain or cramping
* Acid reflux and heartburn
* Acne
* Allergies and food sensitivities
* Anxiety
* Any disorder of the digestive tract
* Autoimmune disorders (rheumatoid arthritis, lupus, Hashimoto's thyroiditis, fibromyalgia, etc.)
* Back pain
* Bad breath, gum disease, and dental problems
* Belching
* Bloating
* Chronic fatigue
* Constipation
* Diarrhea
* Difficulty losing weight
* Diverticulitis/Diverticulosis
* Eczema or psoriasis
* Flatulence
* High cholesterol
* Indigestion
* Irritable bowel syndrome
* Joint inflammation and stiffness
* Lupus
* Nausea
* Poor digestion
* Poor sleep
* Rheumatoid arthritis
* Sinus infections
* Sugar cravings
* Yeast infections or vaginitis (see page 146 for more information on yeasts and candida infections)

There are also many factors that throw off the delicate microbial balance in our intestines, including:

* Alcohol consumption
* Antacid use
* Antibiotic use
* Birth control pills
* Blood sugar imbalances
* Chlorinated water
* Consumption of antibiotic- and synthetic-hormone-containing foods
* Diabetes
* Excessive sugar intake
* Exposure to toxins
* Hypothyroid function
* Immune-suppressing drugs
* Inadequate hydrochloric acid (stomach acid) production
* Mercury amalgam dental fillings
* Multiple sexual partners or sex with an infected person
* Nutritional deficiencies
* Poor diet
* Recreational drug use
* Stress, particularly chronic stress
* Weakened immune system

Top Anti-Inflammatory Essential Oils

While there are many dietary and lifestyle factors that increase inflammation, it is possible to reduce the toll they take on our body. Essential oils, when properly selected, and correctly and consistently used, are among the best natural anti-inflammatories. Here are some of the best:

COPAIBA
(Copaifera reticulata, C. officinalis, C. coriacea, and C. langsdorffii)

One of the most powerful anti-inflammatory remedies on the planet, copaiba is my first choice for addressing inflammation of all kinds. Copaiba originates in the Amazon rainforest, so choose only copaiba essential oil that has been harvested in a sustainable way. In other words, these massive trees should not be cut down to extract their oil;

they should be tapped like maple trees in a way that maintains the health of the tree. Additionally, choose only products that are pure enough for internal use since that is one of the most effective ways of using copaiba essential oil. If using topically on any inflamed areas, apply a drop or two over these areas, diluting it with three parts carrier oil to one part copaiba if you have sensitive skin, and take two to three drops on your tongue up to three times daily to quell systemic inflammation that may be linked to your hormonal imbalances.

FRANKINCENSE
(Boswellia frereana)

Frankincense is both anti-infectious and a potent anti-inflammatory, making it an excellent remedy to address inflammation in the gut. In one study, researchers found that the essential oil showed significant antibacterial action against the three types of bacteria tested, *E. coli*, *Bacillus subtilis,* and *Staphylococcus aureus,* the bacteria that causes the sometimes deadly MRSA (methicillin-resistant *Staphylococcus aureus*) infection. These antibiotic-resistant bacteria are linked with food poisoning and other serious health-damaging infections. Other research in *Letters in Applied Microbiology* journal also found frankincense helpful against *Candida albicans* and *Staphylococcus aureus* infections, which are common infections that play a significant role in gut health and gut microbial imbalances. Fortunately, frankincense is effective against biofilms as well. Biofilms are a thick, potentially health-damaging layer of micro-organisms that secrete substances that help ensure their survival in or on the body. They are usually present in infections that are difficult to eradicate like those mentioned above. Take one to three drops on your tongue or in an empty capsule up to three times daily. Diluted frankincense can also be applied to the skin in areas where inflammation may be an issue, such as over the adrenal glands or thyroid gland, which you'll learn more about in the coming chapters.

GINGER
(Zingiber officinale)

You'll want to add ginger to a lot more foods than just gingerbread to take advantage of its powerful anti-inflammatory properties. Research that compared the anti-inflammatory effects of ginger to those of cortisone and ibuprofen, drugs that are used to treat inflammatory conditions, found that ginger was superior to ibuprofen at reducing inflammatory compounds known as cytokines and was equally effective as cortisone. Unlike cortisone, however, ginger does not have the lengthy list of nasty side effects, such as weight gain and headaches. While the study was conducted on cell cultures created using samples from arthritics, ginger's wide-reaching anti-inflammatory effects make it an excellent choice for addressing low-grade, systemic inflammation as well. Pure ginger essential oil can be used internally; it is a bit spicy so you'll want to add it to empty capsules. Like frankincense, it can be diluted in a carrier oil and applied over any area where there is inflammation.

ROMAN CHAMOMILE
(Anthemis nobilis)

A study published in the *Journal of Natural Products* assessed the anti-inflammatory properties of Roman chamomile and found that the herb contains at least one anti-inflammatory compound. Use Roman chamomile aromatically by diffusing it or adding it to skincare or massage blends for topical use.

TURMERIC
(Curcuma longal)

Primarily known for lending color and flavor to curries, this root contains a potent anti-inflammatory known as turmerone. While bright yellow curcumin gets all the press and indeed has anti-inflammatory properties in its own right, turmeric essential oil is a great source of turmerone, which is not found in curcumin supplements and only in small amounts in turmeric powder. Many studies demonstrate turmerone's inflammation-fighting abilities. To reap the benefits of this oil, add two to three drops to an empty capsule and take up to three times daily.

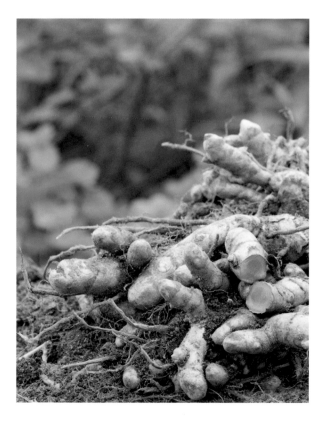

TAKE DOWN THE INFLAMMATION BLEND

I recommend this formula to clients to address underlying inflammation that may be involved with hormonal imbalances.

Yield: 1 capsule

* 1 empty capsule (available in most health food stores)
* 2 drops copaiba essential oil, suitable for internal use
* 2 drops turmeric essential oil, suitable for internal use
* 1 drop frankincense essential oil, suitable for internal use
* Fractionated coconut oil or extra virgin olive oil

Open the capsule. Add the essential oils. Top up the capsule with fractionated coconut oil or olive oil. Take one capsule twice daily as a natural anti-inflammatory.

Top Antibacterial Essential Oils

While many people consider antibiotics the best medicines against bacterial illnesses, bacteria are increasingly becoming resistant to the antibiotics that were intended to kill them. Fortunately, a growing body of research shows that essential oils may be the best-kept secret against a wide range of bacterial infections, from gut bacterial imbalances to urinary tract infections, and others. Unlike antibiotics which indiscriminately kill both beneficial and harmful bacteria, essential oils address the harmful ones only, leaving beneficial bacteria intact. While you can use these oils to treat just about any type of infection, getting underlying gut infections under control is critical to the success of your hormone-balancing regime. Here are some of my favorite antibacterial essential oils:

BASIL
(Ocimum basilicum)

Basil has been shown to have excellent anti-infectious qualities. Research in the journal *Molecules* found that natural volatile oils in basil inhibited multiple drug-resistant strains of *E. coli* bacteria. *E. coli* can cause cramps, diarrhea, and vomiting linked to food poisoning, as well as gut inflammation. According to a preliminary study published in *BMC Complementary and Alternative Medicine*, scientists demonstrated that an extract of basil seeds was even effective in the laboratory against tuberculosis-causing bacteria.

GERMAN CHAMOMILE
(Matricaria chamomilla)

Germany's Commission E, a scientific advisory board to the government, approved German chamomile as a skin treatment to reduce swelling and fight bacteria, as well as a tea or supplement to alleviate stomach cramps.

Researchers assessed the antimicrobial activity of an extract of German chamomile against the fungus *Candida albicans*, which plays a role in oral as well as gut health. This study could help explain German chamomile's reputation for healing dental abscesses and gum inflammation.

CINNAMON
(Cinnamomum zeylanicum)

Cinnamon essential oil is a potent antibacterial. In a study published in *BMC Complementary and Alternative Medicine*, cinnamon essential oil derived from the bark was found to have strong antibacterial activity against several harmful strains of bacteria, including multiple Salmonella strains linked to food poisoning, *E. coli*, *Staphylococcus aureus*, and others. Because it is so strong, you'll want to take one drop in an empty capsule and top it up with olive oil before ingesting.

GINGER
(Zingiber officinale)

According to well-known herbalist and author, Stephen Harrod Buhner, more and more exciting research showcases ginger's potency against viruses and bacteria alike, even when antibiotic or antiviral drugs fail. That's important news as we collectively cope with resistant superbugs. Ginger essential oil can be diluted and applied topically or ingested in an empty capsule.

OREGANO
(Origanum vulgare)

Oregano is a powerful antiseptic thanks largely to the compounds carvacrol and rosmarinic acid. Unlike antibiotic drugs that work only on bacteria, these compounds in oregano fight viruses, fungi, and even parasites like worms as well, making it a well-rounded plant to keep in your natural medicine cabinet and use to maintain a healthy gut. Like cinnamon, oregano is strong so you'll want to take one drop in an empty capsule and top it up with olive oil before ingesting.

ROSE
(Rosa damascena)

It's easy to assume that the delicate scent of rose means it must not have potent antibacterial properties. But, rose is a powerful antibacterial oil that has demonstrated effectiveness against all six bacteria strains it was tested on, including some drug-resistant varieties.

TEA TREE
(Melaleuca alternifolia)

Tea tree (or melaleuca, as it is also called) has been used for centuries for its potent antibacterial action. Research in the *Journal of Antimicrobial Chemotherapy* found that tea tree essential oil was even effective against MRSA, which the researchers attribute to the natural compounds known as alpha terpineol and linalool. Other research published in the *International Journal of Antimicrobial Agents* showed that tea tree oil is effective against *S. aureus* and the biofilms they create. Depending on the type of infection, tea tree oil can be applied to the skin or diffused in the air.

THYME
(Thymus vulgaris)

In a review of thyme, oregano, and basil published in the *Journal of Microbiology and Biotechnology*, researchers found that all three were effective against a variety of bacterial strains. In their assessment of the oils' effects on *E. coli*, the researchers found that both thyme and oregano were the most effective.

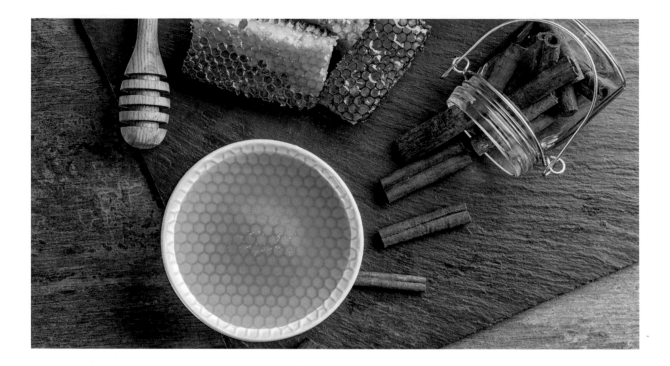

ULTIMATE ANTIBACTERIAL CAPSULE

This is a powerful antibacterial formula I regularly use with my clients.

Yield: 1 capsule

* 1 empty capsule (available from most health food stores)
* 1 drop oregano essential oil, suitable for internal use
* 1 drop thyme essential oil, suitable for internal use
* Fractionated coconut oil or extra virgin olive oil

Open one capsule. Add the essential oils. Top up with fractionated coconut oil or olive oil. Close the capsule. Take one capsule three times daily for the prevention or treatment of infections.

ANTIBACTERIAL CINNAMON HONEY

You'll find this is a great way to reap the benefits of cinnamon and honey, while also being more flavorful, potent, and less gritty than just adding cinnamon powder. You can make a larger batch to store in a small glass jar for up to a year, if desired.

Yield: 1 teaspoon

* 1 drop cinnamon essential oil, suitable for internal use
* 1 teaspoon unpasteurized honey

In a small bowl, mix together the cinnamon and honey until well blended. Enjoy on toast, over oatmeal, or in your favorite dish.

Support Your Overburdened Liver

With over five hundred functions to perform, your liver is one of the most overworked organs in your body and performs more biochemical tasks than any other organ. Some of the liver's many functions include storing vitamins, minerals, and sugars for use as fuel; controlling the production and excretion of cholesterol; and creating thousands of enzymes that control almost every function in your body. It helps your body break down fat, proteins, and carbohydrates, and processes hemoglobin in the blood to allow it to use iron. Most relevant for us, it also maintains balanced hormone levels. No matter what type of hormonal imbalance you're dealing with, it is imperative to support your liver and the many tasks it performs for your body.

Our modern lifestyle monumentally adds to the liver's workload. Your liver must filter any foreign substance that enters your body. That includes alcohol, tobacco, environmental pollutants, food additives, common cosmetic ingredients, household products, pharmaceutical and over-the-counter (OTC) drugs, and caffeine. It must also process internally created substances like the byproducts of metabolizing food and stress; filter excessive amounts of sex hormones; and much more.

The average person consumes fourteen pounds of food preservatives, additives, waxes, colors, flavors, and pesticide residues each year, most of which are hormone disruptors! Guess whose job it is to filter out all those potentially harmful substances? That's right: the liver. Your liver filters all these chemicals, including those that act as potent hormones within the body—all while filtering excessive amounts of hormones. For example, when you pop an acetaminophen tablet to reduce a headache, the liver filters it. Actually, acetaminophen is also one of the worst liver-harming culprits. It can seriously damage your liver's ability to perform its many functions, leaving you feeling less-than-great. When the liver is not functioning optimally, its ability to filter toxic hormone disruptors and excessive hormones suffers.

The liver simply cannot handle the onslaught of toxic chemicals and harmful substances we throw at it. Yes, most of us do so unknowingly, but the liver-damaging effects are the same.

Signs of a Stressed-Out Liver

You don't have to be diagnosed with a serious liver condition like hepatitis, jaundice, or fatty liver to have the signs of a stressed-out liver. Everyone's body is different so you may have only one symptom or health condition, or you may have a handful or more. Here are some things that are linked to reduced liver function or an overwhelmed liver:

* Abdominal bloating
* Alcohol intolerance
* Allergies
* Arthritis
* Asthma
* Bowel infections
* Brain "fog"
* Chronic fatigue syndrome (CFS)
* Colitis
* Crohn's disease
* Depression
* Difficulty losing weight
* Environmental illness or multiple chemical sensitivities
* Fatigue
* Fatty liver
* Fevers
* Fibromyalgia
* Fluid retention
* Gallbladder disease
* Gallstones or gravel
* Gastritis
* Headaches and migraines
* Hepatitis
* High blood pressure
* High cholesterol levels
* Hives
* Hypoglycemia (unstable blood sugar levels)
* Hormone imbalances
* Immune system disorders
* Indigestion
* Irritable bowel syndrome
* Mood swings
* Poor appetite
* Recurring nausea and/or vomiting with no known cause
* Skin conditions like psoriasis and eczema
* Slow metabolism
* Weak digestion
* Weight gain or obesity

Most people are surprised to learn that an over-worked liver can be linked to so many undesirable health symptoms and conditions. Conversely, when you strengthen the liver, you also see improvements in many areas of your health. Essential oils can make a significant difference in improving liver health.

Essential Oils for a Healthy Liver

Most people are familiar with using essential oils for their bath and beauty benefits, but when it comes to liver health, essential oils are among the most powerful medicines available, helping protect and heal the liver and even assisting in weight management issues that accompany liver inflammation. Here are some of my preferred essential oils for a healthy liver:

COPAIBA
(Copaifera reticulata, C. officinalis, C. coriacea, and C. langsdorffii)
Copaiba has powerful anti-inflammatory properties, largely due to its beta-caryophyllene (BCP) content. Research in the *British Journal of Nutrition* found that BCP helps protect the liver against damage in rats. For this purpose, copaiba essential oil is taken internally, usually two drops two to three times daily. Be sure that the essential oil you select is suitable for internal use, and remember to choose a variety that is sustainably harvested through tapping the copaiba trees, rather than chopping down these important rainforest medicines.

FRANKINCENSE
(Boswellia frereana)
The "King of Oils" may be known primarily for its skin and brain health benefits, but that doesn't mean it can't help boost the liver too. Research in the journal *Frontiers in Pharmacology* found that frankincense demonstrated liver-protecting, anti-inflammatory, and antioxidant properties in tests on mice, suggesting that it may be an excellent choice for addressing the free-radical damage and inflammation that often underlies liver issues. It can be diluted for topical use over inflamed areas or specific glands (you'll learn more about them in the upcoming chapters) or a couple of drops can be added to an empty capsule and taken a few times daily to address inflammation.

GERANIUM
(Pelargonium graveolens)
Not just beautiful flowering plants for your garden, geranium also provides a fragrant essential oil that has many healing properties, including stimulating the function of the liver. It can be diluted in a carrier oil and applied topically to the liver region.

HELICHRYSUM
(Helichrysum italicum)
Helichrysum has a lengthy history of use for liver detoxification and stimulation, making it an excellent essential oil to include in your liver-healing repertoire. Dilute the essential oil and apply over the liver, which lies just under the lower right ribs.

LAVENDER
(Lavandula angustifolia)

The liver plays an important role in regulating blood sugar. According to aromatherapy expert and author of *Advanced Aromatherapy*, Kurt Schnaubelt, PhD, lavender normalizes the blood sugar output by the liver. He recommends one or two drops taken internally about 15 minutes prior to a meal to achieve these results.

LEMON
(Citrus limon)

Aromatherapists have used lemon essential oil for many years to help cleanse and protect the liver from harmful free radicals. It can be incorporated into a blend that is diluted with a carrier oil and rubbed onto the liver region a few times daily for a month. The limonene naturally found in lemon essential oil can boost your body's production of glutathione—a critical nutrient in liver detoxification that helps neutralize toxins. Add a drop of lemon essential oil to your water or add a drop to your cooking or baking. It is concentrated so one or two drops is all that is usually needed.

PEPPERMINT
(Mentha piperita)

According to the French aromatherapy tradition, peppermint is beneficial for strengthening and regenerating the liver, making it an excellent choice. To use peppermint for its liver-supporting benefits, take one or two drops on the tongue.

ROSEMARY
(Rosmarinus officinalis)

Rosemary essential oil contains numerous anti-inflammatory compounds that make it an excellent choice for inflammatory conditions, which most are. It is also a powerful antioxidant that fights harmful free radicals. Research in the journal *BMC Complementary and Alternative Medicine* demonstrated potent liver-protecting abilities when administered to rats with liver damage.

TURMERIC
(Curcuma longal)

Turmeric is a powerful natural anti-inflammatory that can help reduce liver inflammation and the weight gain or obesity often linked with it. Research in the journal *Biofactors* found that the spice alleviated inflammation and helped to protect against some of the health-damaging effects of obesity. As you may remember, turmeric contains a potent natural healing compound known as turmerone, which is also a liver cell regenerator and toxin eliminator. Its active ingredient, curcumin, is an incredible anti-inflammatory that may help reduce liver inflammation. Curcumin increases two enzymes that the liver needs to complete the first two phases of the detoxification process that occurs in our bodies on an ongoing basis. It also ensures that phase two can keep pace with phase one. That may not sound like a big deal but some toxins become more toxic if they are only partially broken down in phase one. So, having phase two keep pace is critical to great health.

DR. COOK'S ULTIMATE LIVER HEALER INTERNAL BLEND

This is the powerful liver-healing formula I use with clients in my practice.

Yield: 1 capsule

* 1 empty capsule
* 1 drop copaiba essential oil, suitable for internal use
* 1 drop peppermint essential oil, suitable for internal use
* 1 drop rosemary essential oil, suitable for internal use
* 1 drop turmeric essential oil, suitable for internal use

Add the oils to an empty capsule. Take 1 capsule three times daily.

Tip: As a timesaver, make a large bottle of this essential oil blend and simply add 4 drops of the blend to empty capsules as needed.

LIVER LOVE ROLLERBALL

This blend is a combination of some of the best liver-supporting essential oils in a convenient rollerball format. You can apply it over your liver every night before bed and every day after showering. Your liver is located on the right side of your abdomen, below the lower right ribs.

Yield: 1 (10-milliliter) bottle

* 5 drops copaiba essential oil
* 5 drops frankincense essential oil
* 7 drops geranium essential oil
* 5 drops helichrysum essential oil
* 8 drops rosemary essential oil
* Fractionated coconut oil or carrier oil of your choice

In a 10-milliliter rollerball bottle, add the essential oils, then top it up with fractionated coconut oil and replace the cap. Gently shake until the oils have thoroughly combined.

LOVE YOUR LIVER DIFFUSER BLEND

This is a great liver-healing blend that also has relaxing qualities.

Yield: 1 use

- ❊ 3 drops copaiba
- ❊ 4 drops lavender
- ❊ 3 drops rosemary

Add the essential oils to a diffuser. Diffuse for twenty minutes, three times daily. Continue for at least one month.

LIVER LOVE DIFFUSER BLEND

This blend boosts liver health while also restoring physical and mental energy.

Yield: 1 use

- ❊ 2 drops lemon
- ❊ 4 drops lavender
- ❊ 4 drops rosemary

Add the essential oils to a diffuser. Diffuse for twenty minutes, three times daily. Continue for at least one month.

LIVER SUPPORT BATH SOAK

Store this blend in a large glass jar so you can enjoy a liver health–boosting bath whenever you'd like. It will last indefinitely.

Yield: 4 uses

- ❊ 4 cups Epsom salt
- ❊ 8 drops rosemary essential oil
- ❊ 7 drops frankincense essential oil
- ❊ 12 drops geranium essential oil

In a 1-quart or 1-liter jar with a lid, mix together the Epsom salt and the essential oils. Replace the lid and shake thoroughly to combine all the ingredients.

Use 1 cup of the mixture in a bath. Soak for at least twenty minutes.

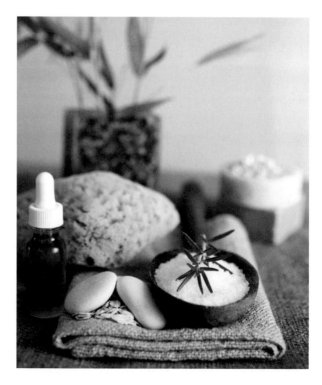

LIVER BOOSTER WHOLE BODY MOISTURIZER

You can gently boost your liver over time simply by adding some essential oils to your favorite moisturizer and using it on a regular basis.

Yield: 1 use

* 1 drop geranium essential oil
* 1 drop lavender essential oil
* 1 drop rosemary essential oil
* A dollop of your favorite toxin-free, unscented moisturizer (see page 41 if you would like to make your own)

Add the essential oils to the moisturizer. Mix well. Apply regularly after showering.

LOVE YOUR LIVER WATER

Boost the liver-healing benefits of the water you drink by adding lemon essential oil.

Yield: 1 serving

* 1 drop of lemon essential oil, suitable for internal use
* 2 cups water

Add the drop of lemon essential oil to the water. Stir and drink.

LIVER-HEALING AROMATHERAPY COMPRESS

It may be hard to imagine that a cloth compress with carefully selected essential oils could have any effect on your liver, but it can. Your skin is your body's largest detoxification organ and can absorb many of the things you put on it. That means an aromatherapy compress placed over your liver can have huge healing benefits. The compress delivers oils that are absorbed directly into the blood that feeds this organ, helping it cleanse your body. This recipe calls for castor oil, which is available in most health food stores.

Yield: 1 application

* 3 layers unbleached or uncolored cotton flannel (approximately 12 x 6 inches each)
* ½–1 cup castor oil
* 5 drops any of the following essential oils: peppermint or lemon
* A dry cloth (to place between the cotton flannel and the hot water bottle)
* Hot water bottle or electric heating pad

Stack the three layers of cotton flannel on top of each other. On the top layer, pour the castor oil so it is saturated but not dripping. Add your selected essential oils. Place the compress, oil side against your skin, over your abdomen, just below your lower right ribs on the front of your body.

Place a dry cloth over the flannel sheets. Top with the water bottle or electric heating pad. Lay back and relax for 30 to 60 minutes.

Balance Your Blood Sugar Levels

Are you trying to have your cake and eat it too? And doughnuts, cookies, and candy bars as well? If your sweet tooth seems to be in charge of you and your eating habits, it may be time to tame it once and for all.

The timing couldn't be better. A growing number of studies link sugar consumption to many serious health concerns. A study published in the *Journal of the American Medical Association* conducted by researchers at the Harvard School of Public Health found that the calories from added sugar in a person's diet are associated with a significantly increased risk of death from heart disease. The study also found that the higher the added sugar intake (particularly from sweetened beverages), the higher the risk of weight gain, obesity, type 2 diabetes, abdominal fat, and high blood pressure.

It will probably come as no surprise that ongoing regular consumption of sugar can cause a wide range of hormonal imbalances. It can impair healthy insulin production and the body's ability to correctly use it to produce energy. Without sufficient energy, the body's ability to perform its many functions becomes impaired, while causing a domino effect of imbalanced hormones as other glands attempt to address the stressful situation.

Do You Have Excess Insulin?

The following are some of the symptoms and conditions linked to excessive amounts of insulin:

* Abdominal fat ("love handles")
* Age spots
* Alzheimer's disease
* Andropause or erectile dysfunction (in men)
* Burning feet at night (usually in bed)
* Cataracts
* Cellulite
* Cravings for breads, pastas, or sweets
* Excessive hair growth on the face or chin (in women)
* Fatigue after eating
* Fatty back of arms
* Fatty liver disease
* Gout
* Heart disease
* High blood pressure, cholesterol, or triglycerides
* Infertility
* Irregular menstruation
* Light brown or dark brown skin patches (usually found on the neck or underarm, known as acanthosis nigricans)
* Low blood sugar (hypoglycemia)
* Menopausal symptoms
* Overweight or obesity
* Poor concentration or memory
* Puffy face or bloating in the face
* Reduced vision
* Sagging breasts
* Skin tags
* Sleep deprivation or disruption
* Type 2 diabetes
* Wrinkling

5 Easy Ways to Regulate Blood Sugar Levels

There are many ways to regulate blood sugar levels both for healthy individuals or those who are trying to address diabetes. Of course, you should be monitored by a physician if you have diabetes because you may find that you'll need to adjust your medication.

1 Eat more fibrous foods like legumes, nuts, seeds, and whole grains that help to stabilize the release of sugar into the bloodstream.

2 Eat protein at every meal. See page 44 for plant-based protein options.

3 Skip the soda; drink water instead.

4 Eat a meal or snack every two to three hours and avoid skipping meals.

5 Scrap hidden sugars: Sugar is hidden in many surprising places, including bread coatings, hamburgers, canned fish, packaged meat and poultry, table salt (shocking but true), luncheon meats, bacon, canned meat, bouillon cubes (and therefore soup), peanut butter, cereals, ketchup, cranberry sauce, and other condiments.

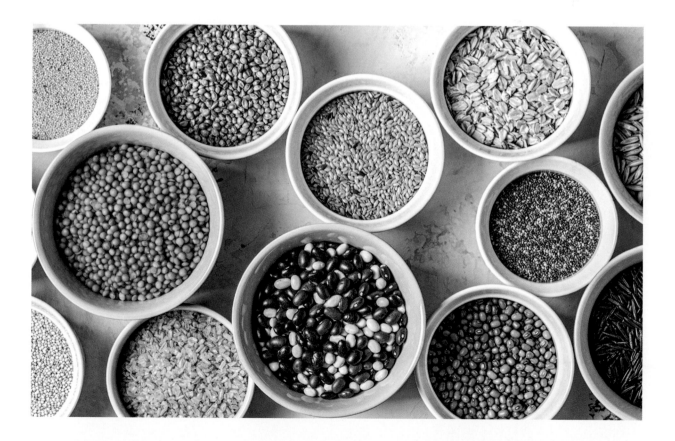

Essential Oils That Help Balance Blood Sugar Levels and Weight

There are many great essential oils that can help you restore healthy and balanced blood sugar as well as a healthy weight. Here are some of my favorites:

CINNAMON
(Cinnamomum zeylanicum)

Cinnamon is not just for sprinkling on lattes. Research in the journal *Lipids in Health and Disease* shows that cinnamon can reduce high blood sugar levels and help regulate other symptoms of metabolic syndrome. Metabolic syndrome describes a collection of symptoms, including abdominal fat, high blood pressure, and abnormal cholesterol and triglyceride levels, as well as high glucose levels. It is often a precursor to diabetes, heart disease, and stroke.

CLARY SAGE
(Salvia sclarea)

While testing of this essential oil for the purposes of blood sugar balancing and weight loss is still in its infancy, one exciting study found that exposure to clary sage essential oil helped to regulate blood sugar levels similarly to insulin and also demonstrated that it had potential to assist with weight loss.

GINGER
(Zingiber officinale)

Researchers have found that ginger significantly lowered blood sugar levels and also helped regulate blood cholesterol levels, suggesting that the herb may offer potential as a natural diabetes treatment in humans.

GRAPEFRUIT
(Citrus × paradisi)

Research shows that rats that consumed grapefruit essential oil gained less weight, and had a reduced risk of excess insulin and less inflammation than rats that had no grapefruit essential oil. Other studies showed that exposure to grapefruit essential oil decreased appetite, food intake, and body weight. Exposure to the scent, such as through diffusing, for fifteen minutes a few times weekly, had a noticeable effect.

JUNIPER
(Juniperus communis)
Research shows that juniper contains potent anti-obesity compounds. While there is little research testing the oil for its weight loss benefits, diffusing it or adding it to a massage blend or moisturizer may help you reap its benefits.

 ### PEPPERMINT
(Mentha piperita)
Drinking water with a drop of peppermint essential oil (see Endurance Boost Water on page 69) boosts energy, which results in increased exercise endurance, thereby improving your capacity for weight loss. In a study of exercise performance published in the *Journal of the International Society of Sports Nutrition*, researchers found that the addition of peppermint essential oil to the water of athletes improved their performance. They found that the study participants who drank the peppermint-infused water were able to exercise longer before feeling exhausted.

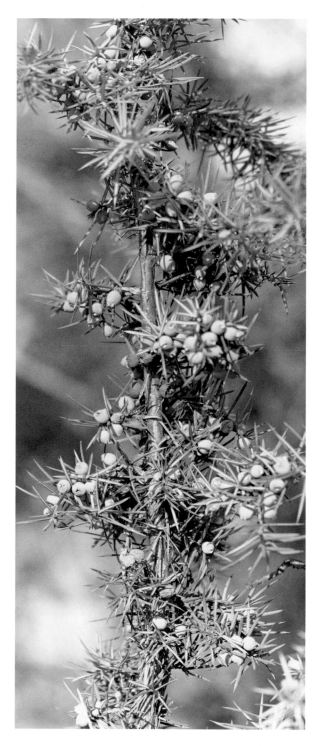

Avoid Hormone-Disrupting Toxins

Every day, we are exposed to countless toxins in our personal care products, cosmetics, cleaning products, laundry soap, fabric softeners, scented candles, air fresheners, and other products in routine use. While it may be tempting to assume that government agencies have studied and verified the safety of these chemicals, few have ever had any safety testing.

Here are some of the most common hormone disruptors to which you may be exposed, as well as where you'll find them, so you can start eliminating them from your life. You'll be surprised to learn that the smell you attribute to soft, clean clothes, or freshly washed hair is probably the result of toxins in your laundry soap, fabric softener, shampoo, or other personal care product that can throw off your delicate hormonal balance. Read the ingredients on all of the products you buy, whether they are for your personal care regimen, cleaning products, air fresheners, or others. If there is no ingredient list, it is likely because the company has something to hide. Choose products whose manufacturers have a commitment to full-disclosure and natural ingredients, or make some of the recipes that you'll find later in this book.

Common Hormone-Disrupting Toxins in Your Daily Life

While we are exposed to thousands of different toxins, here are some of the most common ones that can impact your hormones. Avoiding them as much as possible is one of the keys to great hormonal health.

Alpha-terpineol This chemical is used in cleaning products like laundry soaps and fabric softeners, and has been linked to disorders of the brain and nervous system, loss of muscle control, depression, and headaches.

Benzyl alcohol Found in many laundry products like fabric softeners, benzyl alcohol has been linked to headaches, nausea, vomiting, dizziness, depression, as well as disorders of the brain and nervous system.

BHA and BHT Butylated hydroxyanisole (BHA) and butylated hydroxytoluene (BHT) are common preservatives in personal care products and cosmetics, particularly lipsticks and moisturizers. BHA has been linked to cancer and hormone disruption, liver and thyroid problems, as well as a male hormone disruptor that interferes with reproduction.

DEA Diethanolamine (DEA) and related compounds are used to make cosmetics creamy or to adjust the acidity level in personal care products or cosmetics. They can cause liver or thyroid gland issues.

Dibutyl Pththalate Used as a solvent for dyes in many personal care products and cosmetics, dibutyl pththalate (DBP) is a serious reproductive hormone and fertility disruptor. In a study published in the journal *Environmental Research*, scientists found that prenatal phthalate exposure had a negative impact on the reproductive function of men, including reduced semen volume. In another animal study published in the medical journal *Reproductive Toxicology*, scientists found that even short-term exposure to dibutyl phthalate significantly disrupted ovarian functions in female animals. Sadly, these chemicals are commonplace in products like cosmetics, perfumes, colognes, soap, hair products, skincare products, and deodorants.

Fragrance or Parfum Approximately 3,000 chemicals are lumped together under the classification of "parfum" or "fragrance." Even cosmetics that are listed as "fragrance-free" or "unscented" usually contain these toxic fragrances as well as chemical masking agents to hide the smell of the products in which they are used. They are linked to hormonal issues, migraines, depression, and more. You'll find them in body care products, cosmetics, perfumes, colognes, laundry detergents, and fabric softeners.

Linalool Found in many laundry products, this synthetic chemical (not the natural kind found in some essential oils) can disrupt brain communications and is linked to depression.

Parabens Parabens are preservatives commonly used in beauty products, and are well-established hormone disruptors. Parabens in cosmetics may be linked to hormonally-related breast cancers.

Propylene glycol Also a known carcinogen, propylene glycol is toxic to the immune system, is linked to allergies, accumulates in the body, and irritates the skin, eyes, and lungs.

Siloxanes Siloxanes are silicone-based cosmetic ingredients that are also used in building sealants and lubricants. They are toxic to the reproductive system, potentially harming fertility; high amounts may even cause uterine tumors.

Volatile Organic Compounds Dr. Gaurab Chakrabarti, MD, PhD, at the Philadelphia-based biotechnology company Solugen, conducted a study measuring the amount of volatile organic compounds (VOCs) released by common household products. VOCs are gases that enter the air through the routine use of many products, including paints, cleaning products, pesticides, body care and personal care products, and many more. VOCs have been found to have a wide range of health effects, including cancer and damage to the liver, kidney, brain, and central nervous system.

While many of these products contain harmful amounts of VOCs, the company found that the inappropriately-named "air fresheners" were by far the worst culprits, releasing 697.6 milligrams of VOCs per year per household, based on average use. Shockingly, this was more than the VOCs from some ant and roach insecticides. That amount was followed by disinfecting wipes (358.2 mg), insecticide sprays (238.2 mg), face cleaners (105.4 mg), general glass cleaners (104.2 mg), wood cleaners (52 mg), and dish soap (21.7 mg). Most people choose low- or no-VOC paints, but are unknowingly filling their homes with toxic VOCs through cleaning and personal care products.

Eliminate Hormone-Disrupting Chemicals from Your Home

We are exposed to more synthetic chemicals in our food, air, and water than ever before. Sadly, many companies have duped people into thinking their products are safe so consumers might not even be aware of the nasty toxins they inadvertently invite into their homes. Here are eight simple ways to eliminate hormone-disrupting chemicals from your home:

1. Skip the So-called "Air Fresheners": Whether they come in ozone-depleting aerosol cans, plug-in, candle, or spray bottle formats, the vast majority of so-called "air fresheners" have been found to contain dangerous phthalates. These nasty chemicals are linked to abnormally developed male genitalia, poor semen quality, low testosterone levels, and other reproductive issues. And, if that isn't bad enough, they typically contain lighter fluid, acetone (the same ingredient that makes up nail polish remover), liquefied petroleum gas, and a dizzying array of other toxic ingredients that increase the risk of breathing disorders.

2. Reduce the Amount of Plastic You Use: Just because you may have switched to BPA-free (Bisphenol-A) plastic doesn't mean you are safe from the damage plastics can cause. Many manufacturers removed BPA from their plastics, replacing the toxic ingredient with equally damaging compounds with estrogenic activity (EAs). These synthetic chemicals pose a threat to human health, and to children in particular, increasing aggression, damaging the immune system, and wreaking havoc on hormones. Switch to stainless steel or glass water bottles, food storage containers, and other household items.

3. Stop Heating Food in Plastic Containers in a Microwave Oven: The heat increases the leaching of the plastic's toxic ingredients into the stored food. In research published in the journal *Environmental Health*, both BPA-free plastic and BPA-containing plastic were found to have estrogen activity, which means that they can throw off the delicate hormonal balance when they contaminate our food or water.

4. Make the Laundry Switch: Most commercially available laundry detergents and fabric softeners are loaded with harmful, and even cancer-causing, ingredients. Just because the government has deemed the amounts used as safe doesn't mean that the ingredients were tested for safety. Here's a sampling of the chemicals in most laundry products: alpha-terpineol (linked to disorders of the brain and nervous system, loss of muscle control, depression, and headaches), benzyl acetate (linked to pancreatic cancer), and pentane (linked to headaches, nausea, dizziness, fatigue, drowsiness, and depression).

5. Stop Cooking with Teflon-coated Cookware: Teflon, also known as perfluorooctanoic acid or PFOA, has been linked to cancer, birth defects, and heart disease. Simply choose Teflon-free cookware options.

6. Start Filtering Your Drinking Water: Our tap water now contains a myriad of toxic ingredients, including lead, chlorine, fluoride, and even sometimes prescription medications and hormones. Choose the best-quality water filter you can afford. Even a simple pitcher model will likely be better than nothing at all (assuming you choose one that isn't loaded with all sorts of chemical ingredients).

7. Add a Water Filter to Your Showerhead: While you're picking up a water filter, be sure to add one to your showerhead. There are many affordable options that simply attach to a standard showerhead. Most of our water now contains chlorine, which we breathe in and absorb through our skin in the shower; however, most showerhead filters remove chlorine.

8. Choose Sustainable and Healthier Flooring Options: Carpets contain a whole host of toxic ingredients, including the carcinogen formaldehyde. Vinyl plank flooring and linoleum can off-gas chemicals for years after they are installed. Choose sustainably harvested wood, tile, bamboo, cork, or another type of healthy flooring option when you are renovating or building your home.

ALL-NATURAL ALL-PURPOSE CLEANER

Here's a natural alternative to harmful, hormone-disrupting chemical cleaning products.

Yield: 1 gallon

* ✱ 1 gallon hot water
* ✱ ½ cup liquid castile soap, available in most health food stores
* ✱ 10 drops thyme essential oil

Combine all ingredients in a spray bottle. Shake before using. Use within six months.

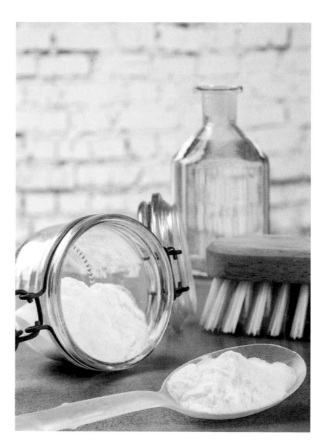

LEMON TEA-TREE
ALL-PURPOSE CLEANER

This variation of the all-purpose cleaner recipe above can tackle any cleaning job. While you can make this cleaner in advance, using hot water helps increase the effectiveness of the cleaner.

Yield: 2½ cups

* 5 drops lemon essential oil
* 5 drops tea tree essential oil
* 5 drops thyme essential oil
* 2 cups hot water
* ½ cup white vinegar

Add lemon, tea tree, and thyme essential oils (about 5 drops each) to 2 cups of hot water and ½ cup white vinegar.

NATURAL PRODUCE WASH

This fruit and vegetable wash will remove waxes and any other residues on your produce.

Yield: 2 cups

* 1 cup apple cider vinegar
* 1 cup water
* 10 drops lemon essential oil

Combine all ingredients in a spray bottle. Spray on fruits and vegetables and let the wash sit for a minute before rinsing. Shake before using. Use within six months.

NATURAL HARDWOOD
FLOOR CLEANER

This blend works well with any type of hardwood flooring.

Yield: Approximately 1 gallon

* 1 gallon hot water
* ½ cup white vinegar
* 3 drops orange essential oil

Combine all the ingredients in a large bucket or container. Use the solution to wipe and mop your floors as needed.

NATURAL MILDEW CLEANER

Mold and mildew don't stand a chance against thyme and tea tree essential oils.

Yield: 2 cups

* 2 cups water
* 30 drops melaleuca tea tree essential oil
* 30 drops thyme essential oil

Combine all ingredients in a spray bottle. Spray on mold or mildew and allow to dry. Repeat as necessary. Shake before using. Use within six months.

LAVENDER CARPET DEODORIZER

This simple recipe will keep your carpets smelling fresh.

Yield: 1 cup

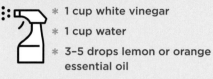

* 5 drops lavender essential oil
* 1 cup baking soda

Combine the lavender essential oil and the baking soda. Sprinkle the mixture on your carpets before vacuuming it to deodorize them.

NATURAL GLASS CLEANER

White vinegar with a few drops of essential oil is more effective and healthier than chemical window cleaners.

Yield: 2 cups

* 1 cup white vinegar
* 1 cup water
* 3–5 drops lemon or orange essential oil

Mix together. Pour into a spray bottle. Shake before using. This cleaner lasts indefinitely.

NATURAL ALL-PURPOSE SCRUB

This natural scrub is a great alternative to toxic commercial varieties.

Yield: Approximately 2 cups

* 2 cups baking soda
* ½ cup liquid castile soap
* ½ cup water
* 5 drops cinnamon
* 5 drops wild orange essential oil

Mix all the ingredients together. Pour into a squirt bottle and shake before each use. Rinse well after use. Use within three months.

NATURAL ROOM DISINFECTANT

Forget toxic air fresheners or deodorizers that are full of hormone-disrupting chemicals. Use this natural room disinfectant instead.

Yield: 2 cups

* 2 cups water
* 15 drops thyme essential oil
* 15 drops tea tree essential oil
* 10 drops oregano essential oil (optional since it has a pungent aroma)

Place all ingredients in a spray bottle. Shake before use. Spray into the air but not directly onto furniture or fabrics to avoid staining. Do not spray directly into the eyes. Keep away from children and pets while spraying.

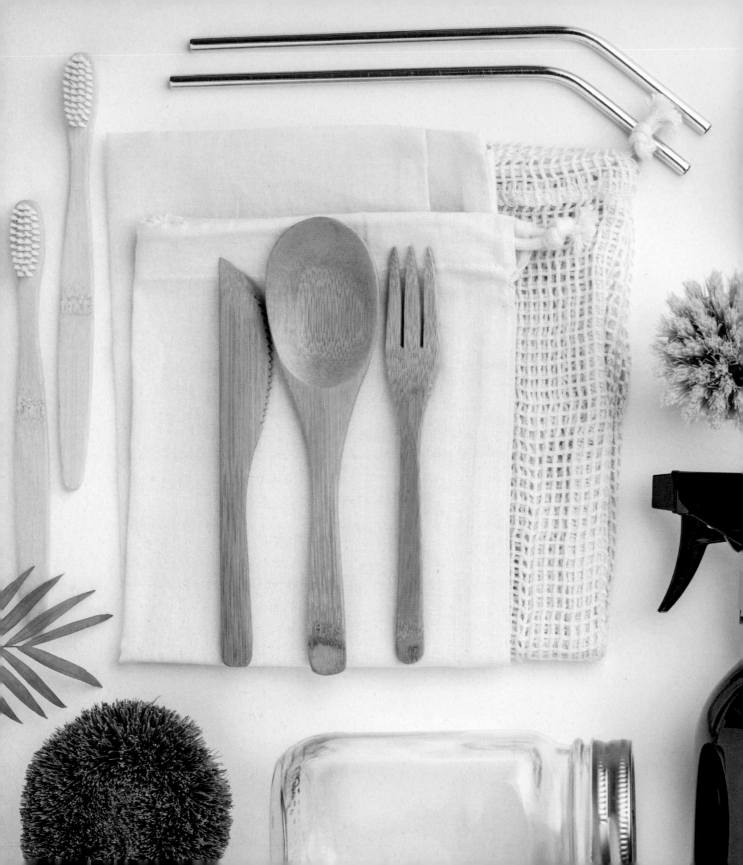

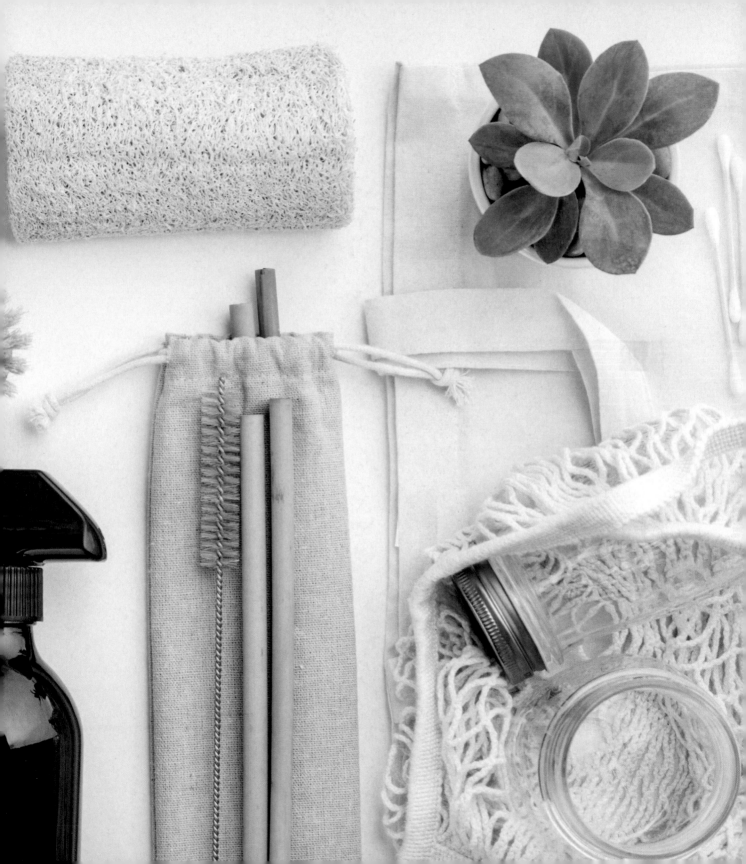

NATURAL LAUNDRY SOAP

Borax, or sodium borate, is a natural, alkaline mineral salt. Like washing soda, borax is also best kept away from children and pets and should never be ingested. Label products made with these ingredients accordingly. Washing soda is found in most health food stores.

Yield: 7 quarts (6.6 L)

* 7 quarts water
* 1 cup soap granules
* ½ cup borax
* ½ cup washing soda (for hard water, double the amount of washing soda)
* 20 drops lavender or lemon essential oil

In a pot, mix 1 quart of water with the soap granules to create a diluted soap mixture. In a clean bucket, add the remaining 6 quarts of water, borax, and washing soda. Add the diluted soap granule mixture and stir until dissolved. Add the lavender or lemon oil. The soap will thicken as it cools. Pour into a large container or jar to store for up to a year.

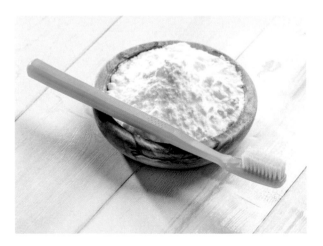

PEPPERMINT REFRESH MOUTHWASH

Skip the synthetic color- and toxic-laden mouthwashes on the market in favor of this natural one.

Yield: 3 ounces

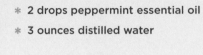

* 2 drops peppermint essential oil
* 3 ounces distilled water

In a small bottle with a lid, mix together the water and the peppermint essential oil. Store the mouthwash in the fridge for up to a week. Shake before each use.

NATURAL TOOTH POWDER

Peppermint and myrrh essential oils in this toothpaste replacement help freshen breath, kill bacteria, and clear sinuses. Myrrh essential oil is highly antibacterial and antifungal. Baking soda restores a natural, slightly alkaline pH balance to the teeth and gums.

Yield: ½ cup

* ½ cup baking soda
* 10 drops peppermint essential oil
* 5 drops pure myrrh essential oil (optional)

Mix the ingredients in a small jar with a lid, cover, and shake well. Use a small amount on a damp toothbrush, and brush your teeth as you would with toothpaste. Keep for up to three months.

FRANKINCENSE ANTI-AGING CREAM

This luxurious moisturizer helps soothe skin, reduce blemishes, and minimize the appearance of wrinkles. Unlike most of the anti-aging creams on the market, this one does not contain petrochemical-based products or chemical preservatives, making it a real treat for your skin. The cream also uses frankincense, one of the most healing essential oils for the skin.

Keep in mind that because it is free of preservatives it doesn't last as long as a chemical-laced commercial product. You may want to use an old blender for this recipe, as the beeswax can leave a film that is difficult to completely remove.

Yield: Approximately 1¾ cups

* ¾ cup sweet almond, apricot kernel, or fractionated coconut oil
* 2 tablespoons shaved beeswax
* 30 drops frankincense essential oil
* 1 cup filtered water

In a small saucepan over low heat, stir almond, apricot, or coconut oil and beeswax together just until beeswax melts. Do not allow oil to become hot. Immediately remove the saucepan from the heat and add the frankincense essential oil.

Pour the water into the blender, cover, and begin blending it on high speed, leaving an opening in the lid. With the blender running, slowly pour the beeswax–oil mixture through the opening in the blender lid. It will begin to thicken after about three-quarters of the beeswax mixture has been incorporated.

Once all the beeswax has been blended, immediately pour the cream into a 16-ounce glass jar or two 8-ounce glass jars. Use it within a month or keep it for up to three months in the refrigerator.

HEALING TEA TREE OINTMENT

This tea tree–infused ointment helps to soothe and disinfect cuts, scrapes, and other wounds after the skin is no longer broken or raw. You may want to use an old blender for this recipe, as the beeswax can leave a film that is difficult to completely remove.

Yield: Approximately ½ cup

* ½ cup extra virgin olive oil
* ⅛ cup grated beeswax
* 30 drops tea tree essential oil

In a small saucepan over low heat, stir the olive oil and beeswax together just until beeswax melts. Do not allow the oil to become hot. Immediately remove the saucepan from the heat and add the tea tree essential oil.

Immediately pour the salve into a 4- to 6-ounce glass jar. Use within a year. Avoid use on broken skin. Reapply as necessary.

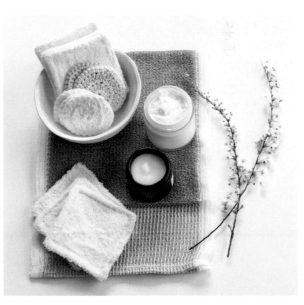

SOOTHING CHAMOMILE CREAM

This silky cream soothes inflammation as it glides across the skin. It is simple to make and doesn't require a lot of ingredients. Because there are no chemical preservatives used, it is a good idea to store this cream in the refrigerator. You will need a medium-size wide-mouthed glass jar or a few small glass jars for storing the lotion. Most healthfood stores sell plain beeswax, which can be shaved with a vegetable peeler. Be sure to avoid other types of wax as they are made of petroleum products.

Yield: 1¾ cups

* ¾ cup sweet almond or apricot kernel oil
* 2 tablespoons shaved beeswax
* 10 drops Roman chamomile essential oil
* 1 cup filtered water

Pour the oil into a heat-safe glass measuring cup and add the shaved beeswax. Set it in a saucepan of water that reaches about halfway up the side of the measuring cup. Heat on the stovetop over low heat until beeswax melts.

Immediately after beeswax melts, remove the pot from the stove. Allow to cool for no longer than a minute or two as the beeswax will begin to harden. Add the Roman chamomile essential oil.

Pour the oil mixture into a blender and blend on high speed with the lid on, leaving an opening in the lid. With the blender running, slowly pour the water through the opening and into oil mixture. It will begin to emulsify and normally thickens after about three-quarters of the water has been incorporated. Continue adding the water until you've incorporated all of it.

Immediately pour lotion into medium-sized wide-mouthed glass storage jars. Use as necessary or desired. Use a spatula to remove any remaining lotion from the blender. Use within three months and store in the fridge.

INVIGORATING LEMON BODY LOTION

One of the best ways to appreciate the invigorating scent of lemon essential oil is to incorporate it into your body lotion or, better yet, make your own lemon body lotion. If you're heading outdoors, it will also help keep mosquitoes at bay. If you're not a fan of lemon, then feel free to use a different essential oil that you prefer.

Yield: Approximately 2 cups

* ¾ cup carrier oil, such as sweet almond oil
* 2 tablespoons shaved beeswax (avoid using other waxes as they are frequently made with petroleum products)
* 30 drops lemon essential oil
* 1 cup filtered water

Pour the oil and beeswax into a small saucepan and heat over low to medium heat until the beeswax melts. Remove from the heat immediately. Allow to cool for 1 to 2 minutes. Add the lemon essential oil.

Pour the water into a blender and begin blending on high speed with the lid on, leaving an opening in the lid. With the blender running, slowly pour the oil–beeswax mixture through the opening and into the water. The mixture will begin to emulsify.

Pour the lotion into one 16-ounce glass jar or two 8-ounce glass jars. Use as desired within three months. The lotion is best kept at cool temperatures to prolong its shelf life. You can also store it in the fridge, if you choose. Avoid sunlight or UV exposure for 12 hours after applying.

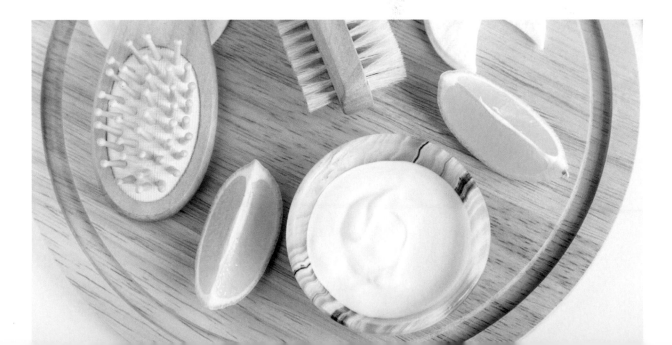

The 10-Day Plan

Hormone-based health issues were among the most frequent conditions for which people consulted my practice. Because hormonal imbalances are usually a symptom, not the cause, of health problems, it is important to get to the root causes behind them. Addressing hormone imbalances usually entails a multifaceted approach involving dietary and life-style modifications, along with targeted natural medicines in the form of essential oils. We'll discuss more about the best essential oils for healing specific types of hormone imbalances in the following chapters.

I developed the following 10-day plan as the foundation for healing hormonal imbalances. While it is designed to be a minimum of ten days, you can, of course, follow it for much longer, and I encourage you to stick with the plan for as long as you can. If you are suffering from long-standing PMS- or menopause-related hormonal symptoms, I encourage you to follow the plan for at least one month, as the body needs time to start cleansing and rebalancing. If you're suffering from a gut condition like a leaky gut or a fatty liver, or something altogether different, you may not completely heal from it within the ten days, but you will be laying the foundation for healing to occur over the longer term. Does that mean you can't have your favorite foods? Of course not. But, I do ask that you stick with the 10-day plan for a minimum of ten days. If

you want to periodically treat yourself to other foods afterward, that's up to you.

By sticking with it for at least ten days, you give your body an opportunity to start eliminating harmful bacteria and toxic material from your gut as well as give your liver a much-needed respite from working so hard. No, that doesn't mean that your liver stops working. It's quite the opposite: feeding your liver more nutrient-dense food and fewer harmful fats and food and reducing the environmental toxins that it has to deal with simply means it can function more efficiently and effectively.

The Plan

If you follow the steps outlined below, you'll soon be well on your way to long-term hormonal health. It may seem daunting at first, but stick with it and you'll quickly realize how easy it can be.

1 Eat a Plant-Based Diet

Plant-based foods are the key to great hormonal health for many reasons. They tend to be higher in water, which is integral to the healthy functioning of every cell in your body. Without adequate water, electrical signals from the brain can misfire. And great hormonal health begins in the brain, where neurochemicals are secreted to control and manage the other hormones in your body. (See chapter 5 to learn more.) Plant-based diets also tend to be high in anti-inflammatory, antioxidant, and other healing phytonutrients that are only found in plant foods. They are also lower in or devoid of (depending on how much meat you eat) animal hormones or synthetic hormones and antibiotics used in the raising of animals for meat. These antibiotics can throw off our delicate balance of beneficial bacteria in our gut.

Plant-based diets tend to be much higher in fiber. Fiber not only ensures bowel regularity, it helps to maintain healthy gut flora populations. It keeps waste matter moving out of the body. This is important not only to prevent harmful substances in the blood but also to ensure the proper absorption of critical vitamins and minerals that are essential to every life function.

Make vegetables the star of every meal. Many people claim they don't like vegetables, to which I say, "You simply haven't tried them the right way yet." No, that doesn't mean battering and frying them. Choose cooking methods that heighten the delicious flavors of vegetables like roasting or sautéeing. You can add roasted beets, asparagus, bell peppers, sweet potato, squash, or other great vegetables to your favorite dishes. Use some imagination. Don't just eat the same pulpy tomatoes and

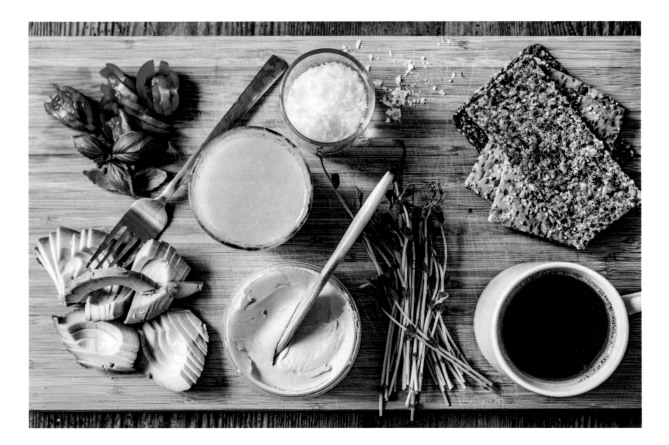

8 Show Your Liver Some Love

There are many liver-boosting foods that offer support and healing to the often-overworked liver, including beets, flaxseeds and flaxseed oil, garlic, leafy greens, lemons, miso, oats, and yogurt (including dairy-free varieties). Add more of these foods to your diet. Ideally, eat them at least two times every day.

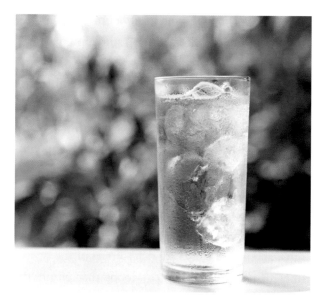

9 Drink More Water

Every cell, and therefore every tissue, gland, and organ, depends on water to perform their many functions. Start every morning with a large glass of water with a drop of lemon essential oil. Drink at least ½ quart or ½ liter (almost the same amount) for every fifty pounds of weight you're carrying, up to about 3 quarts or liters. I know this seems like a lot (because it is!) and you may feel like you're spending your weekend in the bathroom, but water is needed to flush toxins from the body. Without sufficient water, toxins can be absorbed back into the bloodstream, creating a vicious cycle of the liver sloughing off toxins only to have them be reabsorbed into the blood. And try not to drink immediately before or after meals. Freshly made vegetable and fruit juices count toward your total amount of water. Vegetable juices are preferable to water since they contain water along with plentiful amounts of vitamins, minerals, phytonutrients, and enzymes. Freshly made fruit juices also contain these beneficial substances but tend to be high in sugars so they are best consumed in minimal amounts.

10 Eat at least one large green salad daily

No, potato salad or marshmallow-based "salads" don't count as salads. Instead, make your daily salad a gourmet, meal-style salad with a base of leafy greens (real leafy greens like beet greens or kale, not iceberg lettuce), sprinkle some pumpkin seeds or chopped almonds or walnuts over it, add some roasted vegetables, and even some berries or green apple slices. Top it all off with a simple home-made dressing: Mix one part apple cider vinegar to two parts olive oil in a mason jar, along with a pinch of sea salt; some fresh or dried herbs, garlic, or a handful of berries; and a teaspoon or two of pure maple syrup or honey. Vigorously shake the jar after replacing the lid, or blend with a hand mixer until you reach the desired consistency. Don't hold back. Use your creativity to make your salad sing.

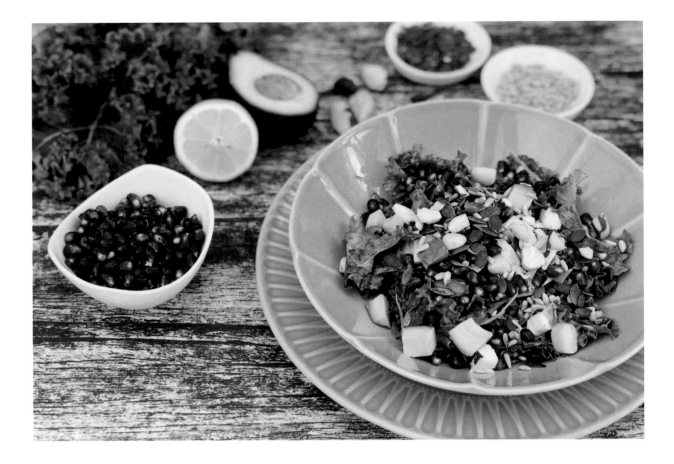

Beginning an Essential Oil Regimen

It's okay to start using any of the essential oils, recipes, or protocols in this book right away and alongside this plan. Actually, the plan works best when you do so.

There's no need to wait to get started. You should begin an essential oil regimen right away based on what seems to be the best fit for the condition you want to address. It's fine to address multiple conditions at once, but be sure not to exceed the maximum amount of oils recommended per day for each recipe or ingest more than twenty drops in a twenty-four hour period, if using essential oils internally.

If you have serious health problems, you'll want to start slowly and work your way up rather than overdo it with too many protocols at once.

If you like, you can keep a journal of your progress and the oils you've opted to take each day. For each health condition you're experiencing, rate the severity of your symptoms on a scale from 1 to 10 with 10 being the worst. Do this prior to starting the plan and then again after you have been following it for a while. This helps to remind you of the improvements you're experiencing, particularly with chronic conditions that may gradually improve.

Simple Ways to Use Essential Oils for Hormone Bliss

You'll find copious recipes and protocols for using essential oils to get incredible therapeutic results for whatever ails you throughout this book, but there are many other ways to benefit from the natural healing power and delightful scents of pure essential oils as part of your daily routine. Here are some great recipes and applications to get you started:

Household

* Add a few drops of antibacterial oils like thyme and cinnamon to your dust cloth before dusting surfaces.
* Add a few drops of lemon essential oil to equal parts of white vinegar and water to clean and disinfect windows and mirrors.
* Add a drop of grapefruit essential oil to the toilet after flushing to freshen the toilet and bathroom.
* Add 5 drops of lavender, wild orange, or grapefruit essential oil to a face cloth and throw it in the dryer with your clothes to give them a fresh, natural, clean scent without the toxic fabric softeners. Use an old face cloth since it may be left with oil stains.
* Put a few drops of peppermint oil on cotton balls around your home to ward off ants, mice, and spiders.
* Put a few drops of cedarwood essential oil on cotton balls in your closet or drawers to keep moths away from your clothes.

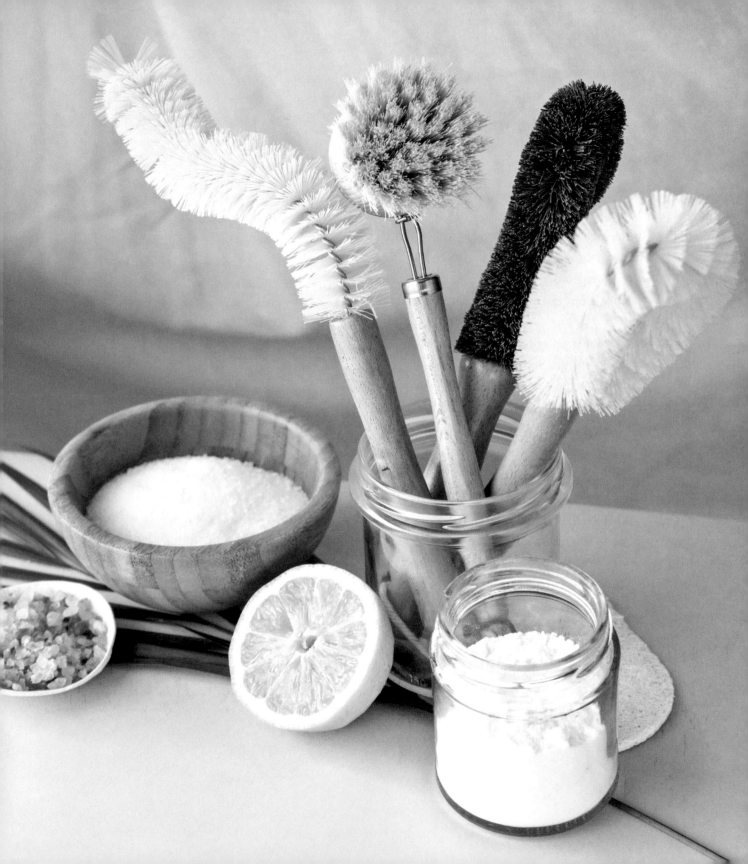

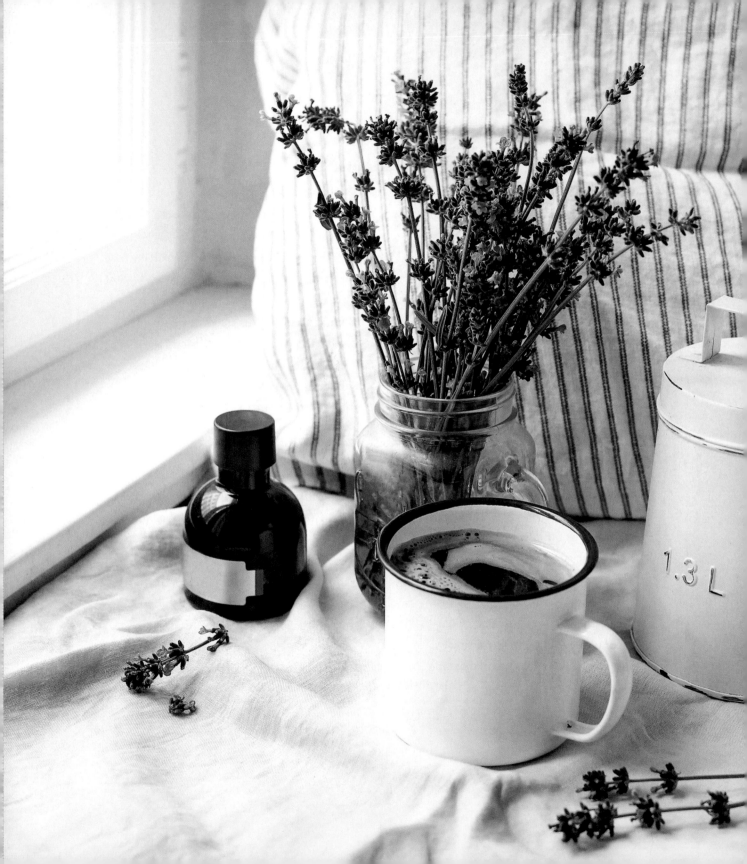

3

Adrenal Rejuvenation
Restore Your Energy and Vitality

D O YOU DRAG YOUR WEARY LIMBS OUT OF BED, need buckets of coffee just to get through the day, and collapse in a heap after dinner? Has balancing work, home, and family responsibilities left you exhausted and overwhelmed? The stresses of our modern life can be too much for your stress glands to handle. The stress glands, primarily known as the adrenal glands, are two small, triangular-shaped glands that sit atop the kidneys and are located in the solar plexus region of the abdomen. They secrete hormones that help us cope with stress, but when the stresses of life become chronic the adrenals can become depleted, leading to adrenal fatigue, or can cause you to alternate between feeling wired and tired.

SUCCESS STORY:
Angela Overcomes Adrenal Fatigue

Angela, a woman in her forties, mother of two children, and a part-time health care aide, explained to me how her doctor had diagnosed her with adrenal fatigue, the depletion of her adrenal glands.

She explained that several years earlier, her husband had been diagnosed with a frequently fatal form of cancer. He had many bouts of chemotherapy and radiation, which had destroyed one of his kidneys, and he simply could not bear the thought of continuing such an invasive and harsh treatment any longer.

The constant fear for his life and the well-being of their young children left her so chronically stressed that her adrenal glands, under constant pressure to produce the hormone cortisol in response, could not handle it anymore. She had tried many of the remedies that her doctor recommended to her. While she saw some improvement, there was not as much as she had hoped.

When I learned that the stress had wreaked havoc on her sleep, I recommended applying lavender essential oil to her feet every night before bed. After only one night of doing so, she awoke with more energy than she had experienced in years. After continuing the practice every night for months, she slowly began to experience greater health and vitality.

Angela uses other great adrenal rejuvenating essential oils as part of her daily regimen, including many of the ones outlined here, but she was impressed that the simple addition of lavender on a regular basis was enough to help increase her energy levels. Once boosted, she began using her newfound passion for essential oils to begin a part-time career teaching others about their many health benefits.

While stress still periodically takes its toll on her adrenals, she feels that she "has gotten more of her life back" with greater energy, the ability to accomplish more throughout the day, and fewer colds and flus that are going around. And, I'm happy to report that her husband, who also uses essential oils as part of his cancer recovery plan, has been cancer-free for over a decade and is one of the longest-living people who have been diagnosed with the rare and severe form of cancer from which he once suffered.

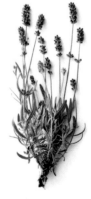

* Drink more than two drinks daily
* Fewer than 7.5 hours of sleep per night
* Food or environmental allergies or hives
* Frequently suffer from colds or flu
* Hair loss
* Heart palpitations
* Infertility
* Irritable bowel or excessive gas and bloating
* Loss of muscle tone in arms and legs
* Love handles or abdominal fat
* Low bone density or osteoporosis

* Low sex drive
* No longer menstruating but haven't started menopause
* Poor concentration or memory
* Puffy or swollen in the face or water retention in the face
* Use of corticosteroids (cortisone, prednisone, etc.)
* Wired at night
* Wrinkled or thinning skin

Essential Oils to Ease Stress

When we think about the causes of stress in our lives, we may simply think of the most common factors, like work-related stress, family worries, and health concerns, among others, but there are many other types of stresses that can strain our adrenal glands. The news these days can wreak havoc on our mood and health. Whether we're watching coverage on politics or reading about the effects of climate change, we are bombarded with a stress-inducing reality that affects our well-being and may even play a role in leaving us depressed and our adrenals feeling overburdened. And, that's not even considering life beyond the screen.

There are other less-considered stresses that can put a strain on our adrenal glands. They include extreme sports, which may seem great at the time because of the "adrenaline junkie" high that they give but over longer periods can deplete the adrenals; perfectionism, which can drive us to excel at all costs; excessive work; temperature extremes; seasonal changes; allergies; and chronic health problems, to name a few.

It's imperative to find ways to boost our outlook and spirits. Essential oils are among the best natural ways to enhance our mood.

BERGAMOT
(Citrus bergamia)

Bergamot is best known for its ability to ease anxiety and lift our spirits, making it an excellent choice to help alleviate stress linked to adrenal fatigue.

CEDARWOOD
(Cedrus atlantica)

The essential oil extracted from cedarwood is a potent natural anti-inflammatory thanks to its anethole content. Cedar helps us relax while also improving mental clarity and focus, making it a great oil to use to deal with the many effects of stress.

CLARY SAGE
(Salvia sclarea)

The essential oil most known for its hormone-balancing effects has been shown in a study published in the *Journal of Ethnopharmacology* to balance brain hormones involved in mood regulation. In another study of menopausal women published in the journal *Phytotherapy Research*, clary sage demonstrated the ability to reduce stress hormones.

FRANKINCENSE
(Boswellia frereana)

Frankincense helps to calm the nervous system, allowing us to better cope with the stresses facing us in our daily lives. In a study published in the *Journal of Psychopharmacology*, the incensole acetate (IA) found in frankincense was found to have antidepressant qualities and regulate the HPA axis by regulating the hormones secreted by the hypothalamus, pituitary, and adrenal glands. Frankincense also contains compounds known as sesquiterpenes, which cross the blood-brain barrier where they can help reset brain chemistry and allow us to better cope with stress.

LAVENDER
(Lavandula angustifolia)

Lavender is perhaps the most widely studied, used, and understood essential oil. And, for good reason: It is a powerful natural remedy with many benefits, including easing anxiety and helping us to obtain a restful and rejuvenating night's sleep, both of which boost our ability to handle stress.

LEMON
(Citrus limon)

The fresh, bright scent of lemon is valuable for more than just cleaning your home; it can help boost your mood. According to a study in the journal *Behavioural Brain Research*, scientists found that lemon was even effective in the treatment of depression.

WILD ORANGE
(Citrus sinensis)

Wild orange or sweet orange essential oil is an uplifting oil that boosts mood and energy levels. Research in the *Journal of Agricultural and Food Chemistry* found that this potent natural remedy is highly effective at resetting the body's natural hypothalamic-pituitary-adrenal (HPA) axis. This axis determines how the hypothalamus and pituitary glands in the brain, as well as the adrenal glands, communicate, helping them work together to achieve hormonal balance. The study found that limonene, a natural compound found in orange essential oil, helped to reduce the damaging effects of chronic, unpredictable, mild stress. Simply inhaling orange essential oil on a frequent basis was enough to improve the effects of stress and restore the HPA axis. Those of us in the natural health profession know that resetting the HPA axis is the key to restoring adrenal gland health, but until now, it has been hard to find treatments that quickly and effectively do this. It will probably come as no surprise that the study also found that frequently inhaling orange essential oil could address depression, sugar cravings, and other symptoms caused by stress.

You can diffuse one or more of the above essential oils in a diffuser to reap their anti-stress effects, or simply inhale the oil several times throughout the day for at least a few minutes each time. Alternatively, add a few drops of the oil to a cloth and sniff it throughout the day, or place the cloth on your pillow to breathe in the scent during the night while you sleep.

Are Your Adrenal Glands Stressed Out?

You've probably already experienced the harsh effects of stress on your body. Stress weakens your immune system, wreaks havoc on your emotions, throws off your metabolism, and impairs your hormone balance. But, when your adrenal glands are stressed out, there are many other signs and symptoms that you may experience, especially those of adrenal fatigue.

Adrenal fatigue is a common condition in which the regular production of stress hormones in response to our highly stressful and fast-paced lives causes the glands to wear down. At first, it may involve the adrenals secreting hormones in excess or at inappropriate times. The natural cortisol biorhythms of higher cortisol in the morning to help us awaken and lower levels at night to help us sleep, may become flipped. You may have high levels of cortisol in the evening rather than in the morning. When that happens, you may find it difficult to get out of bed in the morning and have trouble sleeping at night.

Eventually, chronic stress and the resulting high levels of cortisol that tend to accompany it can cause the adrenal glands to become depleted. Low levels of cortisol are often the result. In this sense, high or low cortisol levels are often opposite sides of the same coin.

Without adequate cortisol, our liver has trouble converting its stored energy, known as glycogen, into glucose—the body's main energy source. Digestion may become impaired, as it often does when the adrenals become depleted. Normally, the foods we eat are broken down into all of the energy and nutrients we need for every cell in our body to perform optimally. Proteins are broken down into amino acids, fats into fatty acids, and carbohydrates into sugars. The remaining food is broken down into their component parts, including vitamins, minerals, phytonutrients, and other nutritional compounds. When our ability to break down proteins, fats, and carbohydrates for fuel becomes impaired or inadequate, we not only have insufficient energy for our tasks but can potentially experience many nutrient deficiencies as well. Over time, this can cause any number of health problems in our bodies, depending on which cells, tissues, glands, organs, and organ systems are affected by these deficiencies.

As the adrenals become worn out further, they may not be able to secrete sufficient cortisol, and you may feel too exhausted to keep up with the demands of the day.

Adrenal Fatigue versus Adrenal Exhaustion

We often call our feelings of fatigue "exhaustion" to more adequately describe the severely low energy levels we feel. As a result, it is common to hear people say that they are experiencing adrenal exhaustion. However, unless they have been diagnosed with the extremely rare, life-threatening disorder called adrenal exhaustion, it is unlikely they have it. This condition involves adrenals that are so severely depleted that they are nearly non-functioning and put a person's life seriously at risk. I'm not talking about the kind of fatigue most people experience. A person with this condition is likely unable to perform most daily functions and struggle even to get out of bed. They are disabled from severe exhaustion. Those with adrenal exhaustion should seek immediate medical attention.

Do You Have Adrenal Fatigue?

Adrenal fatigue can cause a whole host of physical ailments, such as fatigue, poor digestion, sleep disorders, reduced immune system functioning, and elevated blood sugar levels. Here are some of the most common signs that your adrenal glands may be depleted:

* Allergies
* Anxiety or panic attacks
* Arthritis
* Brain fog
* Chronic fatigue syndrome
* Cold sensitivity
* Cravings for sweet or salty foods
* Depression
* Difficulty concentrating
* Digestive complaints
* Excessive fearfulness
* Excessive hunger or low appetite
* Eyes that are sensitive to light
* Fatigue
* Feeling overwhelmed or incapable of coping with life's stresses
* Frequent colds, flu, or other infections
* Gastroesophageal reflux disorder (GERD)
* Impaired memory
* Insomnia or sleep disturbances
* Impatience
* Irritable bowel syndrome (IBS)
* Irritability
* Low blood pressure
* Low libido or interest in sexual activity

* Low stamina or difficulty recovering from exercise
* Menopausal symptoms, including hot flashes, mood swings, or vaginal dryness
* Not feeling refreshed or revitalized by sleep
* Poor concentration
* Premenstrual syndrome (PMS)
* Sensitivity to light
* Slow recovery from illnesses or injuries
* Weak digestion

* Weak immune system or reduced immune function
* Weight gain, weight issues, or weight loss

If you suffer from any health issues, you should visit your physician to rule out any other conditions, but know that most medical doctors aren't versed in adrenal gland conditions unless they are severe, potentially life-threatening cases. Don't be surprised if she or he doesn't recognize the symptoms of adrenal fatigue.

Powerful Adrenal-Healing Essential Oils

While adrenal fatigue can take its toll on your health, you don't have to needlessly suffer. There are many great essential oils that can help you to restore adrenal gland health.

BLACK SPRUCE
(Picea mariana)

Once you experience the scent of black spruce, you'll be amazed that healing the adrenal glands can smell so heavenly. Black spruce is one of the most powerful essential oils to restore the adrenal glands. It can help regulate cortisol levels produced by the glands, and its ability to ease stress helps us to better cope with everyday worries.

GERANIUM
(Pelargonium graveolens)

Geranium is also one of the best natural healers for the adrenal glands. In a study published in *Complementary Therapies in Clinical Practice*, researchers assessed the effects of geranium essential oil on anxiety levels and found that it was significantly more effective than a placebo at reducing anxiety, which is a common symptom of adrenal fatigue.

GINGER
(Zingiber officinale)

The oil extract of gingerroot helps to modulate cortisol levels and normalize blood pressure and heart rate (both of which are intricately involved with adrenal gland health). Additionally, ginger essential oil, when taken internally, can increase your energy and metabolic rate, while also stimulating digestive enzymes to help your body digest proteins, carbohydrates, and fats. People with adrenal fatigue often have trouble with their digestion, which makes ginger essential oil a great choice for both the condition and its symptoms.

PINE
(Pinus sylvestris)

The essential oil of these coniferous trees have been used for many years to help restore adrenal gland health. Research conducted by aromatherapy practitioner and lecturer Shirley Price in her book *Aromatherapy for Health Professionals* found that pine, in conjunction with rosemary, supports the healing of the adrenal cortex. The adrenal cortex makes up the outer portion of the adrenal glands and regulates fat and carbohydrate metabolism, as well as sodium balance in the body, which plays a critical role in healthy blood pressure.

ROSEMARY
(Rosmarinus officinalis)

Like pine, rosemary is a powerful adrenal healer, particularly when used in conjunction with pine essential oil. It contains numerous anti-inflammatory compounds, which, as you learned in chapter 2, is an underlying factor in most health conditions, including adrenal fatigue. Rosemary also contains compounds that boost digestion, which is a common concern for many people suffering from adrenal fatigue.

WILD ORANGE
(Citrus sinensis)

As you learned earlier, wild orange essential oil helps to reset the HPA axis and improve communication between the brain and adrenal glands. This can help us cope with stress and anxiety, while also creating a sense of calmness. Orange oil is also a great all-natural anxiety remedy, a common symptom of adrenal fatigue.

YLANG-YLANG
(Cananga odorata)

Preliminary research in the *Journal of Ethnopharmacology* found that ylang-ylang not only balanced brain hormones linked to anxiety, it also helped to reduce the adrenal gland hormone known as corticosterone, which is involved in stress and immune system reactions.

To use these oils, dilute a few drops of a high-quality essential oil in a teaspoon of carrier oil like fractionated coconut oil or sweet almond oil and rub over the solar plexus region, just below the diaphragm, on a daily basis. Simply diffuse undiluted (neat) pine, rosemary essential oil, or a combination of the two in an aromatherapy diffuser. Inhale the vapors on a daily basis for at least twenty minutes.

HEALING ADRENAL BLEND

When rubbed over the region of the adrenal glands, this powerful blend of oils can help to restore them to health.

Yield: 1 application

* 2 drops black spruce essential oil
* 1 drop pine essential oil
* 1 drop rosemary essential oil
* 1 drop wild orange essential oil
* 2 drops ylang-ylang essential oil
* 1 teaspoon fractionated coconut oil or other carrier oil

Mix the oils together in a small bowl. Rub a small amount over your solar plexus region (the middle of the abdomen just below the diaphragm) at least twice daily for a minimum of one month.

ADRENAL POWERHOUSE ROLLERBALL

In a convenient rollerball form, this adrenal blend can be applied not only on the adrenal region but also the wrists, neck, and other areas to help alleviate stress.

Yield: 1 (10-milliliter) bottle

* 8 drops black spruce essential oil
* 4 drops pine essential oil
* 4 drops rosemary essential oil
* 4 drops wild orange essential oil
* 8 drops ylang-ylang essential oil
* Fractionated coconut oil or other carrier oil

Place the essential oils in an empty 10-milliliter rollerball bottle. Top up with fractionated coconut oil and gently shake until blended. Apply over your solar plexus region and mid-back every morning after showering and before bed for at least one month.

PEACEFUL TIME
ANTI-STRESS DIFFUSER BLEND

When you're feeling anxious or stressed-out, this is a sweet-smelling route to experiencing relaxation and peace.

Yield: 1 use

* 3 drops geranium essential oil
* 2 drops wild orange essential oil
* 2 drops ylang-ylang essential oil

Add the essential oils to a diffuser. Diffuse for twenty minutes, three times daily for maximum benefit.

ADRENAL REJUVENATING BLEND

This blissful blend of oils will make you feel like you're in the forest or a lovely garden while easing the stresses you may be feeling.

Yield: 1 use

* 3 drops pine essential oil
* 3 drops rosemary essential oil

Add the essential oils to a diffuser. Diffuse for at least twenty minutes on a daily basis.

DR. COOK'S ADRENAL REJUVENATION MASSAGE BLEND

This blend features powerful adrenal healers that balance key adrenal hormones like cortisol.

Yield: 1 (100-milliliter) bottle

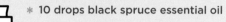

* 10 drops black spruce essential oil
* 5 drops geranium essential oil
* 8 drops pine essential oil
* 5 drops rosemary essential oil
* 5 drops wild orange essential oil
* 100 milliliters fractionated coconut oil or other carrier oil

In a small resealable bottle, add the essential oils. Add the fractionated coconut oil or other carrier oil. Gently shake to blend. Use for any back massage on a daily basis to strengthen the adrenal glands.

MUSCLE TENSION BLEND ROLLERBALL

Many people who suffer from adrenal fatigue also experience sore, tight muscles on a regular basis. Use this blend to help ease tension and achiness.

Yield: 1 (10-milliliter) bottle

* 10 drops wintergreen essential oil
* 6 drops lavender essential oil
* 8 drops peppermint essential oil
* 4 drops coriander essential oil
* 3 drops marjoram essential oil
* 3 drops basil essential oil
* 3 drops rosemary essential oil
* Fractionated coconut oil or other carrier oil

Place all of the essential oils in an empty rollerball bottle. Top up with fractionated coconut essential oil. Replace the top and gently shake to combine all ingredients together. Apply as necessary to sore or tight muscles.

FOREST STROLL TO EASE TENSION DIFFUSER BLEND

This recipe creates one of my all-time favorite blends of essential oils. But don't underestimate it because of its amazing scent—it is also a powerful adrenal healer that helps to ease tension in minutes.

Yield: 1 use

* 4 drops black spruce essential oil
* 2 drops pine essential oil
* 2 drops rosemary essential oil

Add the essential oils to a diffuser. Diffuse for twenty minutes, three times daily for maximum benefit.

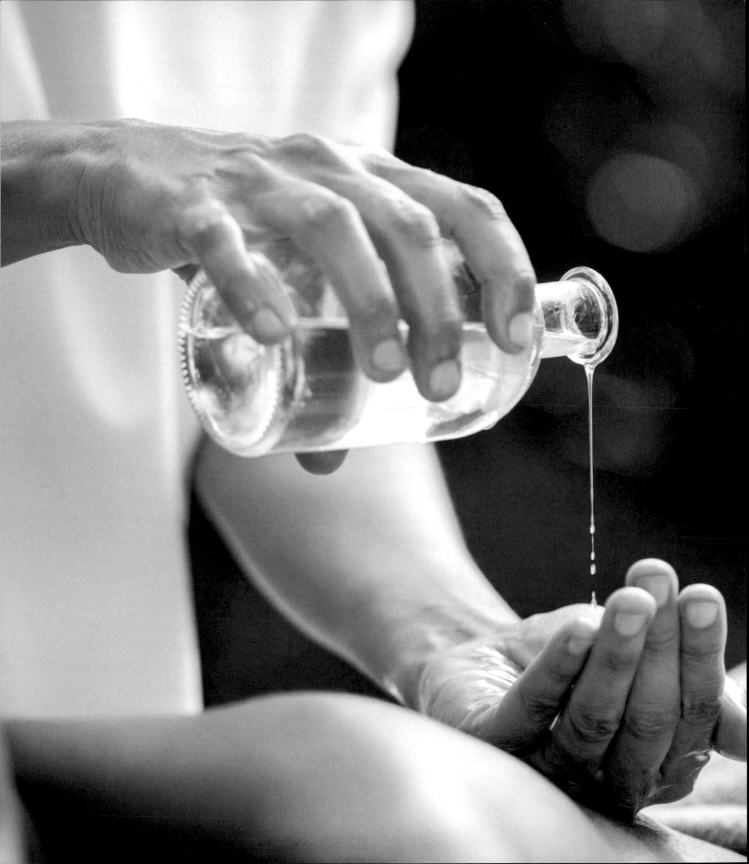

the plant's therapeutic properties into a concentrated form. It has a warming and calming effect on the digestive system and is helpful for most types of digestive issues, particularly nausea and motion sickness. Research found that ginger's digestion-healing properties may be linked to its ability to stimulate saliva, which contains ptyalin, a natural compound that improves carbohydrate digestion, as well as enzymes, which improve digestion. The study achieved these effects through ingestion of ginger extract, but in my experience ginger essential oil offers similar effects. Of course, not all essential oils are suited for internal use so be sure you choose one that indicates internal use on the label and use only a drop at a time.

PEPPERMINT
(Mentha piperita)

Aromatherapists and essential oil experts use peppermint essential oil not only to aid digestion but also to help alleviate food poisoning, gas, vomiting, nausea, digestive upset, and motion sickness. According to research in the medical journal *Food Science and Biotechnology*, peppermint exhibits anti-inflammatory, antioxidant, and even anti-viral effects, all of which play a role in peppermint's wide-reaching therapeutic benefits for digestive complaints. And, due to its anti-viral activity, peppermint essential oil is a great choice for digestive complaints linked with the flu as well.

TARRAGON
(Artemisia dracunculus)

Tarragon is not just a flavorful herb in French cuisine. It can be used medicinally to alleviate indigestion, gas, intestinal spasms, weak digestion, and stomach upset linked to stress.

I have found that using topically, and ingestion of, one or more of the above oils tends to yield the best effects for digestion. Oils like ginger and peppermint tend to be good choices for this purpose.

DIGESTION AID INTERNAL BLEND

This essential oil blend assists with indigestion, nausea, bloating, or other digestive issues. Most people experience improvement within 10–20 minutes of taking a drop or two.

Yield: 52 doses

* 15 drops ginger essential oil
* 13 drops peppermint essential oil
* 10 drops coriander essential oil
* 5 drops tarragon essential oil
* 4 drops fennel essential oil

Combine the essential oils in a small bottle. Gently shake until well combined. Place one drop on your tongue when you feel any digestive discomfort or indigestion. Repeat as necessary, up to 5 drops total per day.

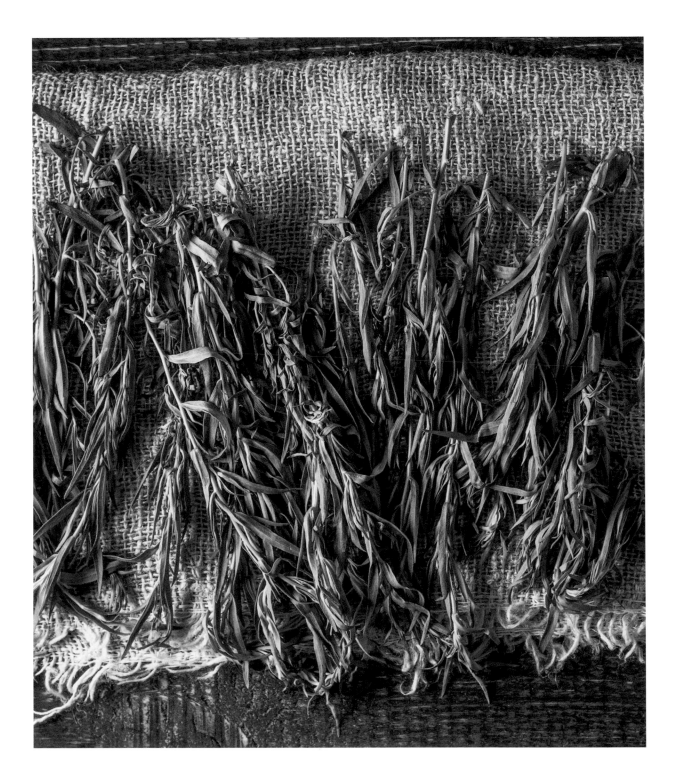

* **Reduce your consumption of sugar and refined wheat products.** They cause your blood sugar to fluctuate rapidly, which can, in turn, cause your adrenals to overreact to the stress.

* **Eat some protein at every meal to help stabilize blood sugar and prevent strain on the adrenals.** That doesn't necessarily mean meat. Some good vegetarian sources of protein include legumes (beans), nuts, seeds, avocado, and quinoa.

* **Supplement with vitamin C.** The adrenal glands are the biggest users of vitamin C in the body. Your body needs vitamin C to cope with stress. The more stress you experience, the higher your vitamin C needs may be. A typical dose to assist with adrenal fatigue is 500 to 2,000 milligram. Do not exceed 2,000 milligram in a single dose.

* **Add pantothenic acid.** Vitamin B_5, or pantothenic acid, is one of the B-complex vitamins that are essential for adrenal gland health. This critical vitamin is naturally present in high doses in the adrenal glands but can become depleted as it manufactures the hormone cortisol in response to stress. A typical dose for combating adrenal fatigue is 1,500 milligram daily, but that amount should come in the form of a B-complex vitamin since the B vitamins work synergistically.

* **Take a deep breath . . .** and then take a few more. Even a few minutes of deep breathing can reduce the stress hormones the adrenal glands secrete. Instead of jumping out of your seat during a traffic jam or other stressful spot, start breathing deeply.

* **Reduce your stress.** I know this sounds impossible to many people. But the truth is that no one else is going to reduce your stress levels for you. While life can be difficult sometimes, it's important to take some time on a daily basis to release stress. Go for a walk, stop and smell the roses (literally, in this case, or at least find some rose essential oil), give a loved one a hug, practice meditation, and get some rest.

* **Try to get at least seven to eight hours of sleep at night.** And if possible, don't wake to a blaring alarm clock since the noise causes your body to release a flood of stress hormones.

* **Exercise regularly but don't overdo it.** Exercise is a valuable release for pent-up stress. Just know your limits and don't overexercise, since extreme activity or extreme sports can stress the adrenals. You may be better off with a gentle stroll, yoga, tai chi, or in severe cases, resting.

Get a Better, Deeper Night's Sleep

Many sufferers of low adrenal function have trouble with sleep: either they need more sleep, or they suffer from insomnia or trouble achieving a deep, restful night's sleep. If you're struggling with getting a good night's rest, there are some simple strategies you can use:

Harness the power of lavender. Alan R. Hirsch, MD, author of *Life's a Smelling Success*, found that smelling pure lavender calmed the entire nervous system in only one minute, helping people to feel more relaxed and sleepier. Sniff some lavender essential oil, flowers, or spray lavender water on your pillowcase (as the oil may stain the fabric). Alternatively, place a drop of lavender on the palms of your hands, inside of your wrists, or on the soles of your feet prior to retiring for bed for a deeper, more restful night's sleep.

Avoid eating at least three hours before bed. Indigestion, bloating, or heartburn can interfere with your ability to fall asleep. Definitely skip the caffeine in the evening.

Practice a regular evening relaxation ritual. Dim the lights, stop working, take a bath, or do something relaxing before bedtime.

Unplug electronic devices or any blue-light emitting appliances like televisions, smartphones, and computers. The blue light can interfere with sleep cycles. If you need a night light, choose one with a red bulb since red light doesn't seem to interfere with the body's ability to fall into a deep state of sleep.

Stop working at least a few hours before bed. Avoid other mentally stimulating activities too close to bedtime.

Go to sleep at the same time each night. Your body will start to adjust to these patterns, helping you to feel sleepy when your bedtime approaches.

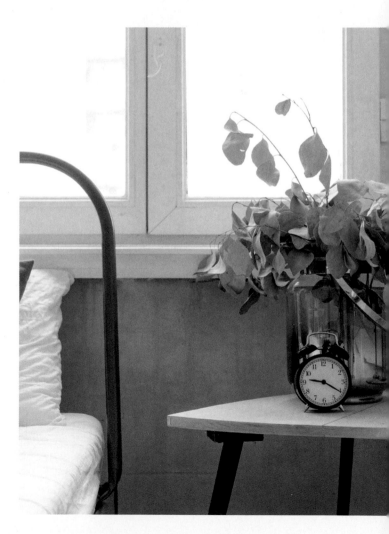

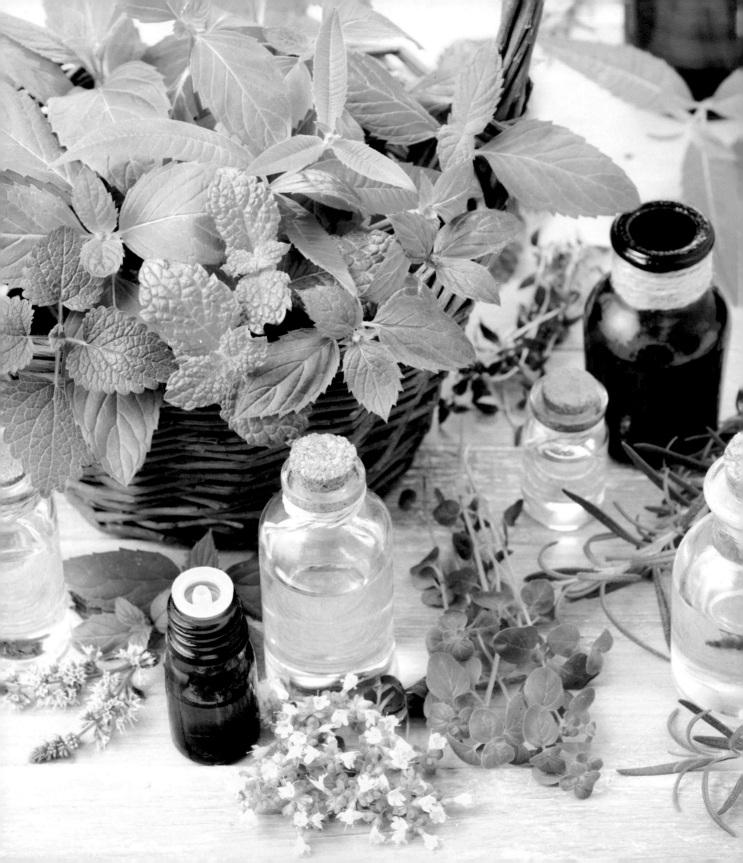

4

Reset Your Thyroid

Balance Your Metabolism
Even When Nothing Else Works

IMAGINE HOW GREAT IT WOULD BE TO SIMPLY REBOOT your body when it starts to malfunction. You could boost your energy; restore a healthy, balanced weight; and reduce feelings of depression. Fortunately, you can do all this by resetting your thyroid gland, the body's main metabolism gland, when it's not operating up to par. While the thyroid is just one small gland in your body, it controls functions throughout it. Once reset, you'll begin to feel better than you have in years.

Some people have no idea why they have low energy, difficulty losing weight, or are feeling cold all the time, never suspecting that a low-functioning thyroid might be behind their suffering. Others seek help from their doctors, but they never conduct all the necessary tests to get an accurate reflection of the thyroid gland's health or the thyroid tests come back normal, making them feel more dejected than ever. Many people suffer from a sub-clinically low-functioning thyroid yet test after test comes back that nothing is wrong, and they are unable to receive any insights from health professionals into how they can address the problem. Still others obtain thyroid test results that show an under-functioning thyroid gland, but the medication prescribed by their doctor does nothing to ease their symptoms. Sometimes people take thyroid medications for years but never feel better.

In this chapter, you'll learn about the gland that underlies many health problems and how you can use essential oils to reset it for great health. You'll discover the Melissa Magic remedy that often resets the thyroid gland in thirty days or less.

Additionally, I'll also share the best essential oils for boosting your metabolism. If you've been suffering with a low-functioning thyroid gland, you'll find natural options here. Before we dive in, let's first explore the thyroid gland and how to know if your thyroid is in need of a boost.

What Is the Thyroid Gland?

The thyroid gland is a butterfly-shaped gland located at the base of your neck, just below the Adam's apple in men. It is sometimes called the metabolism gland because it secretes hormones that are involved in and control metabolic activities taking place in every cell of your body. Thyroid hormones are involved in countless bodily functions: they regulate metabolism, heart rate, cholesterol levels, weight, energy, skin and hair texture, bowel functions, menstrual regularity, organ function, fertility, mood, memory, and many other processes.

Thyroid Hormones 101

There are four main thyroid hormones that work collectively to balance many of the processes I mentioned above. Some are secreted by the thyroid gland while other hormones are secreted by the pituitary gland, which sits in the brain and controls the function of the thyroid gland. Let's take a quick look at them now.

Thyroid-Stimulating Hormone (TSH): Produced by the pituitary gland in the brain, this hormone directs the thyroid gland's output of the thyroid hormone T_4. A high TSH level may mean that your thyroid gland is not responding to signals from the pituitary. In other words, there may be a communication breakdown between these glands so the pituitary secretes additional TSH in an effort to boost the thyroid gland's activity.

Free T_4 (also known as thyroxine): T_4 is the hormone that the thyroid gland produces after receiving instructions from the pituitary gland through TSH. It is the primary form of thyroid hormone found in the bloodstream. This hormone acts as a feedback system to the brain. If levels of T_4 are low, this signals the pituitary gland to make more TSH to tell the thyroid gland to kick it up a notch. Most doctors only test for this hormone, but even normal levels of T_4 don't tell the whole story about the health of the thyroid gland.

Free T_3 (also known as triiodothyronine): Once the thyroid gland makes T_4, it is converted to T_3 in the cells of the body, provided the body has sufficient nutrients and the capacity to do so. T_3 is the thyroid hormone that influences metabolism of all of your cells, tissues, and organs. Similar to T_4, T_3 acts as a feedback mechanism to let the pituitary gland know when it is time to make more TSH, which in turn tells the thyroid gland to increase its production of hormones.

Reverse T_3 (rT_3): If you are under a lot of stress or suffering from a deficiency of the trace mineral selenium, your body may increase its levels of rT_3. When rT_3 levels are high, it usually indicates a low-functioning thyroid gland.

The Effects of Stress on Your Thyroid

When you experience stress, your body may decrease its thyroid function as a way to preserve energy to deal with the stressor. While that may have been helpful for our ancient ancestors who needed to flee a tiger in the jungle on occasion, our less serious but more frequent stressors and severe and chronic stress levels can seriously impact our thyroid health.

As you learned earlier, most of the T_4 in your body is normally converted into T_3, while a small amount is converted into reverse T_3 to balance your system. However, chronic stress can cause our bodies to convert excessive amounts of reverse T_3, thereby slowing metabolism and causing a host of other potential problems. Chronic stress is also linked to excessively high and low levels of the stress hormone cortisol, which can cause hypoglycemia (low blood sugar) or hyperglycemia (high blood sugar). If these blood sugar levels continue to fluctuate over time, they can lead to low thyroid function as well. An increase in the stress hormone cortisol can disrupt the communication of the hypothalamus, pituitary, and thyroid glands as well, causing the communication between the brain and thyroid to further malfunction. This communication is known as the HPT (hypothalamus-pituitary-thyroid) axis.

Does Your Thyroid Need a Reboot?

When your thyroid is not functioning properly, you can feel completely out of sorts. You may gain weight and feel tired and depressed if it is underactive, a condition known as hypothyroidism, or you may lose weight, have trouble sleeping, and experience an irregular heartbeat if it is overactive, which is known as hyperthyroidism.

Do You Have an Underactive Thyroid Gland?

Because the thyroid gland is involved in so many functions in the body, an underfunctioning thyroid gland can result in many possible symptoms. The list on page 81 includes many of the most common ones:

SUCCESS STORY:
Zeina Resets Her Thyroid for More Energy

Zeina, a twenty-one-year-old student working part-time as an administrative assistant to pay for college, came to see me because of low thyroid function. Her condition resulted in weight gain and poor digestion, and she felt cold all the time. She also had unrelenting menstrual cramps that were so severe that they forced her to call in sick for three or four days every month.

Fearful that she would lose her job, and emotionally and physically drained from the monthly pain, she was desperate for help. I put her on the 10-day plan outlined in chapter 2, encouraged her to take one drop of melissa essential oil under her tongue every day, and apply the Thyroid Reset Blend (page 88) three times daily over the front of her neck where the thyroid was located. For her cramps, I advised her to apply my PMS Blend (page 124) to her abdomen two to three times daily every day and instructed her to significantly cut back on sweets.

She came back to see me in a month, astounded that she had more energy, had lost six pounds without trying, had experienced fewer bouts of indigestion, and her cramps had been almost non existent even after years of suffering from horrible pain.

She expressed her shock and dismay that her medical doctor hadn't recommended such an effective remedy at any point during her visits with him. I explained to her that, sadly, while most medical doctors are open to the use of essential oils, few have received any training in the use of the oils and therefore cannot recommend them. Those who use them frequently only have a cursory knowledge of their use and simply don't know which ones to recommend.

She came back to see me a few months later indicating that her digestion was much better and that her monthly periods had come and gone with virtually no pain or discomfort. The improvements had motivated her to stick with the regimen I had given her. She reported that she was experiencing much more energy and had enrolled in natural medicine studies to help others with their suffering using the natural approach that had been so effective for her.

Regardless, Zeina was thrilled with the outcome and was amazed at just how powerful essential oils had proved to be.

* Constipation
* Depression
* Digestive problems, including low stomach acid (hypochlorhydria)
* Dry, itchy skin
* Excessive amount of sleep needed to function during the day
* Fatigue
* Hair falls out easily
* Hypersensitivity to cold weather
* Increased vulnerability to colds and viral or bacterial infections or a lengthy recovery time during infections
* Loss of the outer portion of the eyebrows
* Low body temperature
* Morning headaches that improve as the day progresses
* Muscle cramps while resting
* Poor circulation and numbness in feet and hands
* Slow wound healing
* Swelling or edema, especially in the face
* Thin or brittle hair
* Weight gain or overweight, even on a diet

A low-functioning thyroid gland can also be linked to many female health concerns, including:

* Breast cancer
* Endometriosis
* Miscarriage
* Ovarian cysts
* PMS
* Postpartum depression
* Uterine fibroids

Don't worry: just because you have the symptoms of a low-functioning thyroid gland doesn't mean that you are destined to suffer from breast cancer or another serious health disorder. Remember, it is not necessary to have all of the symptoms above to have hypothyroidism, but if you have any of the ones above, you should consult a doctor.

What about Testing Your Thyroid?

According to the American Association of Clinical Endocrinologists, there are an estimated 27 million people suffering from thyroid disease while 13 million of those cases of thyroid dysfunction go undiagnosed every year. That's astounding. Why are nearly half of the people suffering from thyroid disease doing so without a diagnosis or adequate treatment? There are a number of possible reasons. Some people aren't going to their doctor for assessment and treatment. Those who make an appointment come across blood tests that inadequately detect hypothyroidism in most people. Plus, everyone has different thyroid health needs, and some people may function perfectly fine outside the ranges of what constitutes "normal" thyroid function, while others may be within the range of normal test results and still have hypothyroidism.

Additionally, many doctors only test levels of thyroid-stimulating hormone (TSH) and T_4 even though the other hormones listed on page 78 are equally important to the overall health of the thyroid gland. Testing solely for TSH may mean that doctors miss many people who are suffering from low thyroid function. The latter is an inactive form of thyroid hormone that needs to be converted to a different form before it can be used by the body.

If you haven't been tested for thyroid function yet, ask your doctor to test for TSH, free T_3, free T_4, and thyroid antibodies, since it is highly unlikely that most medical doctors are testing for all four items. Obtaining all four tests will give a more accurate picture of the health of your thyroid gland.

You can also conduct a basal temperature test to assess your thyroid function. The name may make it sound more complex than it actually is, but I've included the full instructions on page 83 to make it easy for you.

What Causes Hypothyroidism?

There are many reasons the thyroid gland stops functioning properly. Here are some of the factors behind a poorly functioning thyroid.

1. The immune system can sometimes attack the thyroid gland, causing what is known as an autoimmune response. This is particularly true in the case of Hashimoto's disease (see page 85).

2. The pituitary gland fails to communicate properly with the thyroid gland. When the pituitary gland doesn't send the hormone TSH to signal the thyroid gland to manufacture thyroid hormones, the thyroid won't make them.

3. The body lacks the ability to convert T_4 into T_3. Even if sufficient T_4 is manufactured by the thyroid gland, it may not convert properly to the active form of T_3, which is the form of thyroid hormone that influences cells, tissues, and organs in the body.

4. There may be dietary nutritional deficiencies. When there aren't sufficient amounts of nutrients such as vitamins, including A, B_2, niacin, B_6, B_{12}, C, and E; amino acids, such as tyrosine; or minerals, such as zinc, iodine, or selenium, the body lacks the building blocks it needs to produce thyroid hormones. Without sufficient construction materials, imagine what your home would look like. It might be missing part of the foundation or part of a roof. You can understand how critical having the right materials is.

5. According to some experts, excessive amounts of fluoride from drinking water and toothpaste can inhibit the thyroid gland from functioning properly.

6. Exposure to some pesticides used on lawns, golf courses, or indoors, or found in our water supply can decrease thyroid function.

7. Exposures to the chemicals polybrominated biphenyls, carbon disulfide, or perchlorate found in water, occupational exposures, or elsewhere, have been linked to decreased thyroid function. Perchlorate is also frequently used in dry cleaning.

8. Overconsumption of soy foods and beverages, particularly those that are unheated or unfermented, can decrease the activity of the thyroid gland.

9. Overconsumption of goitrogens—compounds found in some plant foods that can disrupt normal thyroid function—can also play a role in thyroid health. Goitrogens are primarily found in raw cruciferous vegetables including Brussels sprouts,

Conducting a Basal Temperature Test

Because the thyroid gland reflects the body's metabolic rate and heat is generated during metabolism, assessing basal temperature, or resting body temperature, as it is also known, can give clues regarding the function of the thyroid gland. You should not use a basal temperature test as a replacement for a proper medical assessment, but it can help you determine whether you may have a thyroid imbalance.

1. Shake down a thermometer until the mercury falls below 95 degrees Fahrenheit, if you're using an older thermometer. Place it by your bed at night when you're ready to go to sleep.

2. Upon waking and before getting up (yes, even to use the bathroom), place the thermometer under your armpit for 10 minutes. Digital thermometers may automatically stop before that. Try to lay in bed as still as possible during this time. Rest and close your eyes. Don't get up until after the 10 minutes have passed.

3. Record the temperature, time, and date.

4. Conduct the same test for at least three mornings at the same time each day.

A healthy resting temperature ranges between 97.8 to 98.2 degrees Fahrenheit or 36.6 to 36.8 degrees Celsius. Natural fluctuations can occur during menstrual cycles. If you are menstruating, perform the test on the second, third, and fourth days of the menstrual cycle. Post-menopausal women or men can conduct the tests any days of the month.

If your temperature is consistently lower than the range indicated above for at least three days, this may be an indication of hypothyroidism. Conversely, if your temperature is consistently higher than this, you may have hyperthyroidism or an infection. If you have a higher temperature than the range above, you should see a physician to rule out the latter possibility.

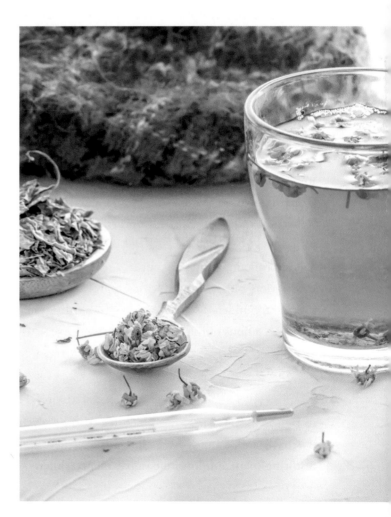

Essential Oils for an Underactive Thyroid Gland

As you learned above, inflammation can be a factor in thyroid gland health. In chapter 2, you read about how inflammation almost always begins in the gut. When it comes to long-term thyroid health, it's imperative to begin by addressing the gut. If you haven't already begun using the anti-inflammatory oils that address inflammation in the gut, refer back to chapter 2. In the meantime, we'll also explore some of the anti-inflammatory essential oils that can help alleviate inflammation in the thyroid itself.

FRANKINCENSE
(Boswellia frereana)

An all-around anti-inflammatory, frankincense also boosts oxygenation of the glands and tissues when applied topically. It has been found in the journal *Scientific Reports* to be particularly anti-inflammatory when used in conjunction with myrrh. Research in *Letters in Applied Microbiology* journal also found frankincense helpful against *Candida albicans*, which is often a factor in thyroid health issues. (To learn more about candida infections, see page 146.)

LEMONGRASS
(Cymbopogon flexuosus)

Lemongrass essential oil is a powerful natural anti-inflammatory oil that also has anti-fungal properties, making it a good oil to use if you're suffering from a candida overgrowth that is common among those with thyroid conditions. Research found that the oil lived up to its reputation for quelling inflammation and destroying fungi.

MYRRH
(Commiphora myrrha)

Myrrh has a lengthy history of use for its potent anti-inflammatory effects and is best paired with frankincense. You can experience its beneficial effects by applying the diluted oil directly over the thyroid gland in the front of the neck to reduce any inflammation in the gland itself. A drop or two taken a few times daily in an empty capsule for at least a month can reduce gut inflammation that may be at the source of thyroid issues.

ROSE GERANIUM
(Pelargonium graveolens var. roseum)

Rose geranium produces not only a lovely scent but also a powerful essential oil that has been found in research to be a highly effective anti-inflammatory. It may also help to alleviate anxiety linked to low thyroid function.

MELISSA
(Melissa officinalis)

Melissa essential oil is one of the best for resetting the thyroid gland. In addition to being anti-inflammatory, melissa has the added value of being anti-viral as well, which may prove beneficial in the treatment of thyroid conditions. Some medical thinkers are increasingly considering the possibility that thyroid conditions may have a viral link. While the topic is still controversial, it warrants consideration as a possibility, particularly since there are some great anti-viral essential oils that could offer tremendous benefit if a virus is playing a role. In a study published in the medical journal *Endocrine*, scientists found a higher incidence of the Epstein-Barr virus among children with autoimmune thyroid conditions. That doesn't prove the link, but it can't hurt to consider using anti-viral essential oils as part of your thyroid program given the safety of essential oils when they are used correctly.

While most oils have some degree of the anti-inflammatory effects, frankincense, myrrh, and rose geranium are among the best ones to apply directly to the front of the neck where the thyroid sits. Keep in mind that a single inhalation or application of the oils will not fix an imbalance, but with regular use and diligence, they may help to restore an underactive thyroid gland. That doesn't mean that you should discontinue your medications and use essential oils as a replacement. However, you may be able to get your doctor to reassess your hormones and medication levels to see if they need to be adjusted after regular use.

DR. COOK'S POWERFUL THYROID PROTOCOL

Rub this convenient-to-use essential oil blend over the front of your neck every day to transform your thyroid health.

Yield: 1 (10-milliliter) bottle

* 10 drops frankincense essential oil
* 8 drops lemongrass essential oil
* 5 drops myrrh essential oil
* 7 drops rose geranium essential oil
* Fractionated coconut oil or other carrier oil

Add the essential oils to an empty 10-milliliter rollerball bottle and top up with fractionated coconut oil. Replace the rollerball top and cap. Gently shake until combined. Roll over the front of the neck and gently massage the oil into the area, three times daily for at least a month. For optimal results, follow with Melissa Magic for the Thyroid (see below) for optimal results.

MELISSA MAGIC FOR THE THYROID

It may seem too simple to be effective, but I've seen melissa essential oil transform thyroid health in people who stick with it.

Yield: 1 dose

* 1 drop melissa essential oil

Place one drop of melissa essential oil on your tongue and hold it to the roof of your mouth for one minute. Repeat daily for at least thirty days.

DR. COOK'S THYROID RESET BLEND FOR AN UNDERACTIVE THYROID

True melissa can be quite costly, but it's worth every penny. Having said that, if it isn't in your budget, leave it out. If the oil you buy is cheap, it's probably because it isn't actually made from melissa but lemongrass, which does *not* have the same thyroid-boosting properties.

Yield: 1 (10-milliliter) bottle

* ✳ 8 drops frankincense essential oil
* ✳ 8 drops melissa essential oil (optional if your budget doesn't permit the addition of this more costly oil)
* ✳ 8 drops myrrh essential oil
* ✳ 8 drops rose geranium essential oil
* ✳ Fractionated coconut oil or other carrier oil

Place the essential oils in an empty 10-milliliter rollerball container. Top up with fractionated coconut oil. Shake gently until combined. Roll the blend over the front of your neck twice daily.

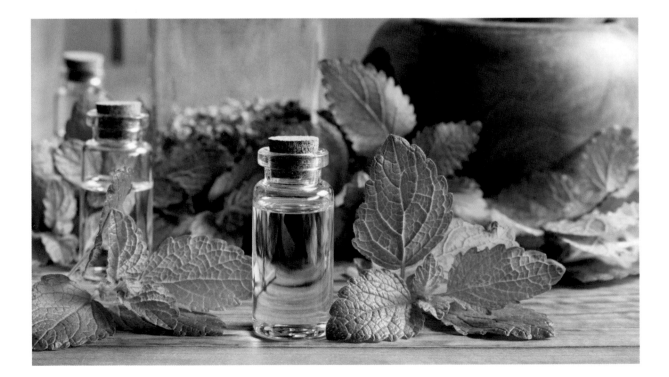

Essential Oils to Boost Your Metabolism

There are many common health issues linked to thyroid imbalances, particularly a low-functioning gland. They include weight gain and a sluggish metabolism, weak digestion resulting in indigestion and other digestive disturbances, as well as thinning hair. In addition to using essential oils to rebalance thyroid hormones and the underlying inflammation often linked to it, you can use essential oils to boost your metabolism. Smelling your way thin may sound too good to be true, but exciting research shows that certain scents trigger weight loss.

LEMON
(Citrus limon)

According to a study published in the journal *Experimental Biology and Medicine*, the scent of lemon (the real stuff, not the synthetic ones added to many commercial cleaning products) activates the nerves in fatty deposits to increase the rate of fat-burning and suppress new weight gain. You can also use lemon topically. To create a massage oil or use lemon with sensitive skin, dilute three to five drops of lemon essential oil in one teaspoon of carrier oil. Avoid sun exposure or UV light for up to 12 hours after using the oil on the skin as lemon essential oil can make the skin more photosensitive during that time frame.

CYPRESS
(Cupressus sempervirens)

Other research at the Department of Nursing at the Wonkwang Health Science College in South Korea found that abdominal massage with specific essential oils reduced belly fat in post-menopausal women. The scientists divided women into two groups: one group used only grapeseed oil while the other group used a blend of grapefruit, lemon, and cypress oils. Study participants massaged their own abdomen twice daily for five days each week and continued for the duration of the study, which was six weeks. The women who used the citrus–cypress blend had significantly less abdominal fat at the end of the study. Their waist measurements dropped significantly and they also experienced an improvement in their body image compared to the control group. While the study only examined post-menopausal women, it is probable that men would experience similar effects as well.

GRAPEFRUIT
(Citrus × paradisi)

Other research published in the journal *Experimental Biology and Medicine* might explain some of the impressive weight loss results of using grapefruit essential oil. In this study, researchers found that grapefruit essential oil activates key nerves to increase fat burning and halt weight gain.

Looking for More Help?

* Thinning hair is a common symptom of thyroid conditions. To discover which oils can help, see page 158.

* Many people who suffer from low thyroid function also deal with poor digestion and indigestion as well. The oils listed on page 69 can help soothe these symptoms.

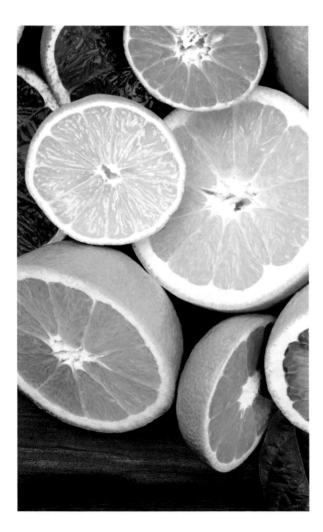

ABDOMINAL FAT-BURNING MASSAGE BLEND

Research has found that the following essential oils can be effective at reducing abdominal fat when applied to the abdomen on a regular basis.

Yield: ¼ cup (60 ml)

* 5 drops grapefruit essential oil
* 5 drops lemon essential oil
* 5 drops cypress essential oil
* ¼ cup (60 ml) fractionated coconut oil or other carrier oil

Add the essential oils and fractionated coconut oil to a glass bottle with a lid. Replace the lid and gently shake until the ingredients are blended together.

Massage a small amount of the oil into your abdomen using large circles starting above your belly button and working outward toward the left side of your abdomen. Perform this massage once or twice daily, or at least five times weekly.

NOTE: Avoid using the blend just prior to sunlight exposure since grapefruit and lemon essential oils can cause slight photosensitivity. Wait at least twelve hours before sun or UV light exposure. While allergic reactions are rare, discontinue use if you observe rashes, hives, or other allergic reactions.

Do You Have an Overactive Thyroid Gland?

Hyperthyroidism means that your thyroid gland produces excessive amounts of the hormone free T_4. An overactive thyroid gland is far less common than an underactive one, but it is often linked to Graves' disease, an autoimmune condition in which your immune system attacks the thyroid, and some forms of goiter, an unusual enlargement of the thyroid. Some of the symptoms of an overactive thyroid gland include:

* Brittle hair
* Changes in menstrual cycle not linked to perimenopause or menopause
* Extreme fatigue or weakness
* Increased frequency of bowel movements without making dietary changes
* Irregular heartbeat or palpitations
* Mood swings
* Nervousness, anxiety, or irritability
* Shaking hands or fingers
* Sleep disturbances
* Sudden loss of weight with no known cause
* Thinning skin

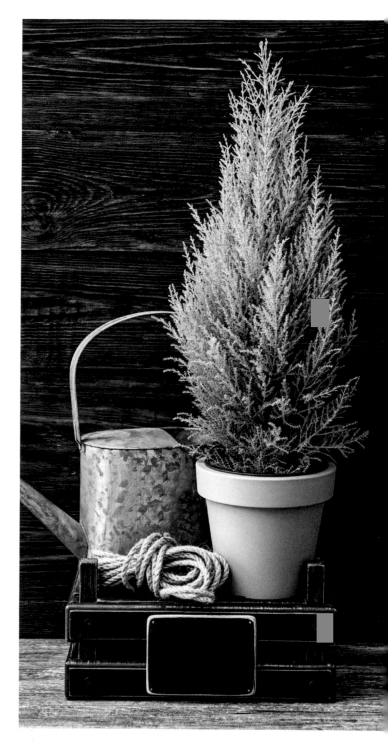

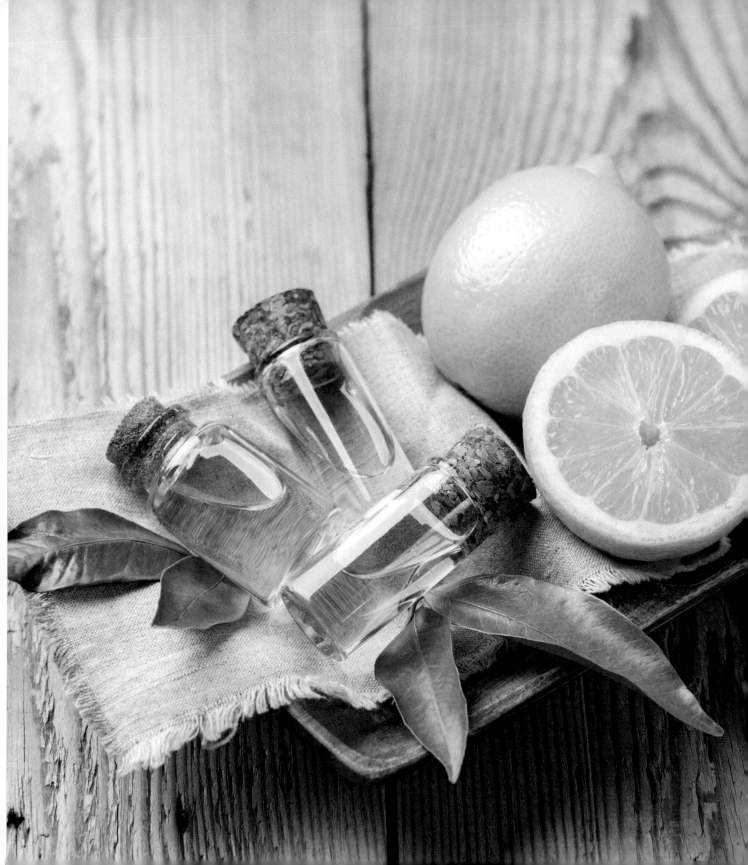

5

Brain Reboot

Harness the Power of Brain Hormones to Transform Your Life

THE BRAIN IS ARGUABLY THE MOST POWERFUL ORGAN in the body. Certainly, when it comes to hormonal health, it takes center stage. It is the command center for the body's other organs, which provide regular feedback to the brain about how they are functioning. The brain uses this feedback to make any necessary adjustments, increasing or decreasing brain hormones so the organs function more effectively. These brain hormones are known as neurotransmitters because they transmit signals between the brain and organs. As a result of this feedback mechanism, the brain impacts our feelings of sadness and depression or joy and happiness. It influences our feelings of anxiety or confidence.

While there are many brain hormones, we'll restrict our exploration to some of the main ones, including dopamine and serotonin. After all, whole books have and could be written on brain hormones alone.

Dopamine: The Reward Hormone

Often called the "pleasure chemical," dopamine is a naturally occurring brain chemical that helps us to feel good and is involved with feelings of reward. The anticipation of a reward, whether a food, drug, money, or something else, can increase levels of this hormone.

Impaired dopamine production is involved in brain disorders like depression and Parkinson's disease, where low dopamine levels are linked with shaky movements. Many addictive substances like alcohol, cigarettes, social media, or even just caffeine, can not only increase dopamine but also have deleterious effects over time.

Things that cause an increase in dopamine become linked with a reward in our minds, while things that cause a decrease in dopamine become linked with disappointment. Dopamine works with serotonin, another neurotransmitter; there's speculation that substances that boost serotonin may also affect dopamine. We'll discuss serotonin more momentarily.

Some of the most common conditions linked to a dopamine deficiency include depression, schizophrenia, and Parkinson's disease.

Do You Have Low Dopamine Levels?

It's important to have sufficient amounts of this brain hormone, as a dopamine deficiency can cause a wide range of undesirable symptoms. These symptoms vary depending on whether you're experiencing the deficiency due to long-term illicit drug use, or diseases like Parkinson's, or something altogether different. Keep in mind that you may have all of these symptoms but not have a dopamine deficiency or, conversely, you may have none of the symptoms and still experience a dopamine deficiency. I've provided the following list of symptoms to help you understand the role dopamine plays in your body, but if you suspect a dopamine deficiency you should still seek medical guidance.

* Aches and pains
* Binge eating
* Constipation
* Cravings for sweets, pastas, breads, or junk or fast food
* Depression
* Difficulty focusing
* Fatigue, especially in the early morning
* Feeling demotivated, or inexplicably sad or tearful
* Feeling hopeless or suicidal
* Frequent pneumonia
* Gastroesophageal reflux disease (GERD)
* Hallucinations or delusions
* Lack of insight or self-awareness
* Loss of balance
* Low self-esteem
* Low sex drive
* Mood swings
* Moving or speaking slower than normal
* Muscle cramps, spasms, or tremors
* Muscle stiffness
* Parkinson's disease

* Poor memory
* Poor tolerance for exercise
* Restless leg syndrome

* Strong desire for excitement or stimulation (foods, gambling, partying, sex, extreme sports, etc.)
* Trouble sleeping or difficulty staying asleep

Essential Oils to Regulate Dopamine

Essential oils are showing tremendous promise in dopamine regulation. Here are some of the best oils in this regard:

BERGAMOT
(Citrus bergamia)

A study published in the medical journal *Current Drug Targets* found that bergamot, as well as lavender and lemon, were effective for depression. In this study the researchers found that the oils stimulated the brain to release two brain hormones that play a role in this condition—dopamine and serotonin.

CLOVE
(Eugenia caryophyllata)

In one study published in the *Journal of Medicinal Food*, researchers found that clove essential oil (as well as a few other essential oils, most of which are difficult to obtain) demonstrated effectiveness in restoring brain dopamine functions. It may even hold promise in the treatment of drug addiction, as dopamine function is typically impaired after lengthy illicit drug use.

GINGER
(Zingiber officinale)

Ginger is best known and widely studied for its anti-inflammatory effects. Because brain diseases (like countless other illnesses) are linked to inflammation, it is no surprise that anti-inflammatory herbs like ginger can be helpful. Research published in the medical journal *Neurology* found that ginger not only reduces the inflammation linked to brain disease, it may be helpful in the prevention or treatment of disorders like Parkinson's. Since brain inflammation can be a factor for brain hormone impairment or full-blown brain disease, no discussion on brain health would be complete without mentioning ginger's anti-inflammatory effects. But there may be other reasons to love ginger: research published in the journal *Neurochemical Research* found that a compound found in ginger prevents the reduction of dopamine involved in Parkinson's disease. While most of the research has been done on the herb itself or herbal extracts, it is likely that the benefits extend to the essential oil.

SUCCESS STORY: Josephine Beats Depression

Josephine, age 48, had perimenopausal symptoms of irregular periods and fatigue that sometimes made it difficult for her to run her clothing manufacturing business. Though hesitant at first to tell me more about her situation, she finally shared that she was suffering from depression and felt too ashamed to let others know. Instead, she hid away in her home during her worst depressive episodes.

Josephine had been suffering for years. When she finally had the courage to reach out, I was eager to do everything I could to help her. I asked her to change her diet and lifestyle to the one outlined in chapter 2 and to do so gradually because I was concerned that she would feel overwhelmed if she tried to implement the full plan all at once.

I made a bottle of equal parts frankincense, oregano, rosemary, and turmeric essential oils and asked her to use two drops in an empty capsule and take three times daily with meals. I also gave her a blend of oils to diffuse or to place a drop in her palms and inhale at least three times daily as well. Eager to recover from the dark place in which she was living, she strictly followed my instructions while staying on the medication her doctor had prescribed.

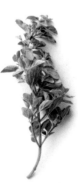

One month later, Josephine came back for a follow-up visit. She indicated that she had experienced significant improvements, e v e n having "good days like [she] remembered having years earlier." She also noticed that when she "cheated" and ate sugary foods she would feel worse soon afterward so she stuck with the low-sugar diet.

While she had made some amazing improvements, I wanted her to feel even better so I encouraged her to continue using the blends of essential oils I had given her. She came back after another month and indicated that she felt so much happier and stronger. While she still had symptoms of depression some days, she was thrilled that she could feel the "dark cloud lifting."

Since experiencing improvement using the oil blends, she also realized that she had stayed in an abusive marriage for decades and finally felt strong enough to face the truth and leave her husband. She came back the following month to report that, while leaving him had been difficult for her, she got through it and was much happier without the constant insults and controlling behavior. She was proud of herself for the first time in many years and felt like she was regaining control of her symptoms, health, and life.

OREGANO
(Origanum vulgare)

A study published in the medical journal *Fundamental & Clinical Pharmacology* found that ingesting a compound called carvacrol, which is primarily found in oregano and thyme essential oils, promoted dopamine production and yielded antidepressant effects in animals. Another study found that ingestion of oregano extract inhibited the deterioration of dopamine, providing enhanced mood and improved behavioral effects. The researchers concluded that oregano "may be effective in enhancing mental well-being in humans."

YLANG-YLANG
(Cananga odorata)

Preliminary animal research published in the medical journal *Phytomedicine* shows that ylang-ylang may be helpful for regulating dopamine levels in males. The study did not achieve the same results in females, but additional research may be helpful in determining whether ylang-ylang could affect women similarly.

Looking for More Help?

* If low dopamine levels have you dragging yourself out of bed each morning, the essential oils on page 97 can help give you an energy boost.

REWARD DIFFUSER BLEND

The ginger, clove, and ylang-ylang help to boost dopamine levels while freshening the air at the same time.

Yield: 1 use

* 2 drops ginger essential oil
* 2 drops clove essential oil
* 3 drops ylang-ylang essential oil

Add the essential oils to a diffuser. Diffuse for twenty minutes, three times daily.

DOPAMINE BOOST DIFFUSER BLEND

Bergamot and ylang-ylang is a heavenly combination that helps to alleviate stress and boost dopamine levels.

Yield: 1 use

* 3 drops bergamot essential oil
* 3 drops ylang-ylang essential oil

Add the essential oils to a diffuser. Diffuse for twenty minutes, three times daily.

DOPAMINE LIFT CAPSULES

I recommend using these capsules to help boost dopamine if you have chronically low dopamine levels or many of the symptoms linked with the shortfall.

Yield: 1 capsule

* 1 drop bergamot essential oil
* 1 drop clove essential oil
* 1 drop ginger essential oil
* 1 drop oregano essential oil
* 1 empty capsule

Add the essential oils to an empty capsule. Replace the capsule top. Take one capsule twice daily with food.

DOPAMINE ENHANCER ROLLERBALL BLEND

Combined in a convenient rollerball, this blend can be kept on an end table, night table, or in your purse to use regularly throughout the day.

Yield: 1 (10-milliliter) bottle

* 12 drops bergamot essential oil
* 5 drops ginger essential oil
* 13 drops ylang-ylang essential oil
* Fractionated coconut oil or other carrier oil

Add the essential oils to an empty 10-milliliter rollerball bottle. Top up with fractionated coconut oil or other carrier oil. Rub on the inside of your wrists and back of your neck three times daily for at least one month.

Serotonin: The Mood, Motivation, and Well-being Hormone

Do you know someone who always seems motivated, energetic, and upbeat about whatever challenges life throws at them? It's not just their good genes, good fortune, or positive thinking that keeps some people so happy. People who have these traits tend to have balanced serotonin levels that help them feel amazing.

Serotonin is a feel-good hormone that helps to ensure we're motivated, have balanced moods, and feel good about life. Low serotonin levels are linked to anxiety, depression, insomnia, and even violent behavior. Serotonin is involved in constricting smooth muscles like those in the bladder, uterus, or gastrointestinal tract. It also helps regulate the body's sleep-wake cycles and the internal clock, social behavior, appetite, digestion, and sexual desire and function. Serotonin even helps to reduce appetite while eating.

You can tap into the power of serotonin to transform your mood, motivation levels, and overall well-being.

Do You Have Low Serotonin?

Low levels of the hormone serotonin are implicated in many conditions, from Alzheimer's disease to depression. As with a dopamine deficiency, you may have all of these symptoms but not have low levels of serotonin or, conversely, you may have none of the symptoms and still experience a serotonin deficiency. Use this list of symptoms to see how serotonin works in your body, but remember, if you suspect a serotonin deficiency, seek medical guidance.

- * Anxiety
- * Bulimia or binge eating
- * Constant hunger
- * Constipation
- * Cravings for sweets, breads, or pastas
- * Depression
- * Difficulty making decisions
- * Feeling wired at night
- * Fibromyalgia
- * Headaches or migraines
- * Inability to sleep in
- * Irritable bowel
- * Lack of sweating
- * Less than 7.5 hours of sleep per night
- * Little motivation
- * Low libido
- * Low self-esteem
- * Nausea
- * Obsessive-compulsive disorder (OCD)
- * Pain or low pain tolerance
- * Poor memory
- * Premenstrual syndrome (with depression and cravings for sweets)
- * Seasonal affective disorder (SAD)
- * Use of corticosteroids (like cortisone, prednisone, etc.)

Essential Oils to Balance Serotonin

While the research on using essential oils for balancing brain neurotransmitters is still in an early stage and certainly more is required, current studies showcase the exciting potential of using essential oils as a way to balance serotonin. Here are some of the best oils for balancing serotonin levels in the brain:

BERGAMOT

(Citrus bergamia)

As you learned earlier, a study published in the medical journal *Current Drug Targets* found that bergamot, as well as lavender and lemon, were effective in the treatment of depression. In another study, researchers found that bergamot essential oil quickly and effectively improved feelings of anxiety. In addition to stimulating dopamine, bergamot also stimulated the release of serotonin. This could play a role in why bergamot is effective in the treatment of these conditions.

LAVENDER

(Lavandula angustifolia)

Known for providing the delightful scent that wafts across the French countryside, lavender also shows tremendous promise in the restoration of healthy serotonin levels in the brain. This could explain its ability to improve mood and reduce anxiety and depression. Research even found that lavender essential oil was about as effective as a common drug used in the treatment of depression. In a study published in the medical journal *Frontiers in Pharmacology*, researchers attribute lavender essential oil and linalool, the naturally occurring compound it contains, to lavender's antidepressant effects. It also helps to regulate serotonin.

OREGANO (AND OTHER CARVACROL-RICH ESSENTIAL OILS)

In a study published in the medical journal *Molecular Biology Reports*, researchers found that carvacrol, which is found in several essential oils, namely oregano, thyme, basil, mint, rosemary, sage, savory, marjoram, hyssop, and lavender, may hold promise in the prevention or treatment of Alzheimer's disease. The preliminary study found that carvacrol was effective at mitigating the damage from chemicals used in mouse models of Alzheimer's disease. The mechanism at work is likely its ability to boost serotonin levels. While the study doesn't yield conclusive evidence that carvacrol-rich essential oils will be helpful in treating Alzheimer's disease, follow-up clinical trials may provide greater insight. However, since carvacrol-rich oils often yield many health benefits and have few, if any side-effects when used correctly, the research warrants consideration. Wild oregano, *origanum vulgare*, has the highest content of carvacrol, containing about 30–87 percent carvacrol, depending on the quality of the chosen essential oil. Thyme, or *thymus vulgaris*, contains up to about 70 percent, again, depending on the quality of the essential oil.

YLANG-YLANG
(*Cananga odorata*)

In a study published in the *Journal of Ethnopharmacology*, scientists found that animals that were exposed to the smell of ylang-ylang essential oil experienced a reduction in anxiety as a result of the oil's balancing effect on serotonin levels. While it would certainly be beneficial to explore follow-up human clinical trials, the advantage of an animal study is that it rules out the possibility of any placebo effect.

Looking for More Help?

* If a serotonin imbalance leaves you susceptible to migraines, seek relief from the oils on page 127.

* Serotonin levels are linked with PMS symptoms, which range from cramps to depression. To learn about the many oils that address PMS, see page 123.

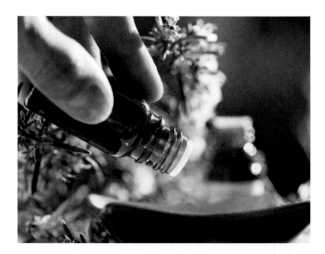

FEEL GREAT DIFFUSER BLEND

A powerful blend of uplifting essential oils, this mixture will uplift your mood and spirit.

Yield: 1 use

* 3 drops basil essential oil
* 3 drops bergamot essential oil
* 2 drops lavender essential oil

Add essential oils to a diffuser. Diffuse for twenty minutes, three times daily.

SEROTONIN-ENHANCING DIFFUSER BLEND

This blend proves that medicine doesn't have to be harsh or unpleasant to be effective. This blend is delightful and effective.

Yield: 1 use

* 3 drops bergamot essential oil
* 2 drops lavender essential oil
* 3 drops ylang-ylang essential oil

Add the essential oils to a diffuser. Diffuse for twenty minutes, three times daily.

SEROTONIN BOOST CAPSULES

If you're suffering from anxiety, depression, or another condition linked to imbalanced serotonin levels, this is a great natural remedy to use, ideally, for at least a month.

Yield: 1 capsule

* 1 drop basil essential oil
* 1 drop mint essential oil
* 1 drop oregano essential oil
* 1 drop thyme essential oil
* 1 empty capsule
* Fractionated coconut oil

Add the essential oils to an empty capsule. Top up with fractionated coconut oil. Replace capsule top. Take twice daily with food.

MOOD MAGIC MASSAGE BLEND

Keep this mood-enhancing blend in a purse, on a night stand, or in your living room to use throughout the day to uplift your mood.

Yield: 1 (10-milliliter) bottle

* 10 drops bergamot essential oil
* 10 drops lavender essential oil
* 10 drops ylang-ylang essential oil
* Fractionated coconut oil or other carrier oil

Add the essential oils to an empty 10-milliliter rollerball bottle. Top up with fractionated coconut oil. Replace the rollerball top and cap. Shake gently to combine. Apply on the insides of your wrists and back of your neck three times daily for at least one month.

Power Your Brain

The brain is involved in every function in your body, every mood you experience, and everything you do in your daily life. Keeping it strong and healthy is important to prevent cognitive decline, maintain a sharp memory, and to prevent or treat brain disorders like anxiety, depression, Alzheimer's or Parkinson's disease, or other brain diseases.

Essential Oils to Boost Overall Brain Health

There are many great essential oils that boost mood, ease depression, and help us cope with the effects of stress or anxiety. Some boost the reward hormone dopamine while others boost the feel-good hormone serotonin. Let's explore some of the best essential oils to boost overall brain health.

COPAIBA

(Copaifera reticulata, C. officinalis, C. coriacea, and C. langsdorffii)

Copaiba's high concentration of beta-caryophyllene gives it highly anti-inflammatory properties and far-reaching healing effects, including on the brain. It holds promise in the treatment of brain diseases like Parkinson's and Alzheimer's, and appears to work against the former disease by protecting the nervous system from damage. A preliminary study published in the medical journal *Biomedicine & Pharmacotherapy* found that copaiba's effects might help protect brain and nervous system cells involved with dopamine production and regulation. In a study exploring the effects of copaiba on brain cells and Alzheimer's disease, researchers found that copaiba provided marked antioxidant, anti-inflammatory, nerve-, and brain-cell protecting abilities. The researchers also found that copaiba prevented the destruction of a brain hormone known as acetylcholine, which is in part linked to the formation of new memories and likely accounts for its brain-boosting and memory-enhancing abilities. A deficiency of acetylcholine has been linked to Alzheimer's disease.

FRANKINCENSE

(Boswellia frereana)

Frankincense contains compounds known as sesquiterpenes, which cross the blood-brain barrier and may help to rebalance brain hormones. The oil also contains a powerful therapeutic substance known as boswellic acid, which has been found in the study *Molecular Neurobiology* to reduce brain and nerve inflammation. As we learned earlier, brain inflammation has been linked to brain health issues like depression.

JUNIPER

(Juniperus communis)

A study in the journal *Neurochemical Research* found that regularly inhaling juniper essential oil could inhibit an enzyme involved in brain diseases and the formation of brain plaques known as beta amyloid, which is involved with Alzheimer's disease. While the research is still in the early stages, this study suggests that juniper essential oil may also hold promise against Alzheimer's disease and dementia. Avoid using if you have kidney disease or while pregnant or lactating.

ROSEMARY

(Rosmarinus officinalis)

This herb doubles as an amazing holiday meal flavoring and a memory enhancer. This long-time reputation for boosting memory likely stems from its ability to increase blood flow to the brain. In studies, rosemary can slow the degradation of acetylcholine. Rosemary has also been found to increase blood flow to the brain, which in turn helps to oxygenate the brain, which could be one of the reasons why it is known to boost memory and concentration.

TURMERIC

(Curcuma longal)

In a study published in the *Journal of Ethnopharmacology*, researchers found that turmeric had a neuroprotective effect, meaning that it protects the brain and nervous system from free-radical or other damage. The researchers studied turmeric in the context of potential natural remedies for the treatment of Parkinson's disease.

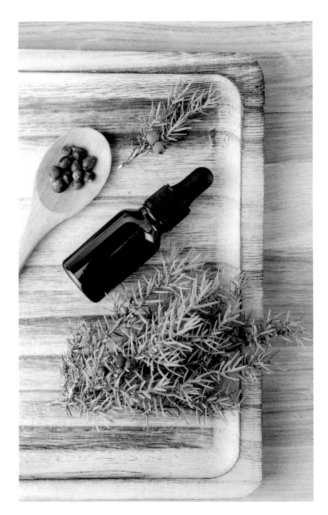

DR. COOK'S BRAIN HORMONE TRANSFORMATION CAPSULES

If you suffer from a poor memory, brain fog, trouble focusing, or other signs of mental stress or decline, this is a powerful formula when used on a regular basis.

Yield: 1 capsule

* 1 drop frankincense essential oil
* 1 drop oregano essential oil
* 1 drop rosemary essential oil
* 1 drop turmeric essential oil
* 1 empty capsule
* Olive oil (optional)

Add the essential oils to an empty capsule and replace capsule top. If you have an irritable stomach, top up with a small amount of olive oil. Start with one capsule daily with food for a week and then move up to two capsules daily for another week, before increasing to, and sticking with, three capsules daily with meals, for at least one month.

MEMORY MAGIC CAPSULES

Another potent blend of natural medicines, these capsules can create a noticeable improvement in memory in just a short amount of time, but I recommend using them for at least a month.

Yield: 1 capsule

* 1 drop copaiba essential oil
* 1 drop frankincense essential oil
* 1 drop rosemary essential oil
* 1 drop turmeric essential oil
* 1 empty capsule

Add the essential oils to an empty capsule and replace the capsule top. Start with one capsule daily with food for a week and then move up to two capsules daily for another week, before increasing to, and sticking with, three capsules daily with meals, for at least one month.

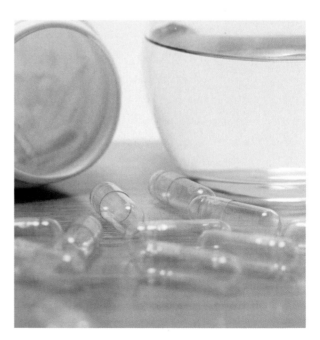

Essential Oils to Ease Depression

Everyone feels down at some point, usually as a reaction to difficult circumstances, but clinical depression goes far beyond that. In such cases, a person experiences a prolonged sadness that is out of proportion with the apparent cause. The physical and psychological symptoms affect a person's capacity to function normally in the world.

Depression is often accompanied by sleep disruption, fatigue, anxiety, mood swings, prolonged lapses of concentration, pain, apathy, decreased sex drive, and suicidal thoughts. Because these symptoms can be attributed to other diseases or conditions and are serious, it is always important to consult a medical doctor for a diagnosis.

Coping with depression can be difficult, but there are natural remedies that may help. Essential oils quickly access the brain via the olfactory system that begins in the nose. Once there, their natural chemical constituents go to work to help restore brain hormonal balance. While there are many excellent essential oils that can help with depression, here are some of my preferred options. Of course, if you're taking prescription drugs, you should continue taking them and be sure to check with your doctor to avoid any possible drug interactions with the essential oils. Additionally, you may need to get your medication modified by your physician if you start to experience improvements from the essential oils, since your doctor may be able to reduce your dose of the drugs.

BERGAMOT
(Citrus bergamia)

Like other citrus oils, bergamot is uplifting, especially when combined with lavender and lemon. A study published in the medical journal *Current Drug Targets* found that bergamot, as well as lavender and lemon, were effective for relieving depression.

CLARY SAGE
(Salvia sclarea)

The essential oil most known for its hormone-balancing effects has been shown in an animal study published in the *Journal of Ethnopharmacology* to balance the brain hormones linked to depression, making it a novel potential treatment for those suffering from the mental illness. In another study of menopausal women published in the journal *Phytotherapy Research*, clary sage demonstrated the ability to reduce stress hormones, which may also be helpful in the treatment of depression.

FRANKINCENSE
(*Boswellia frereana*)

In a study published in the *Journal of Psychopharmacology*, a natural compound found in frankincense, known as incensole acetate (IA), was found to have antidepressant qualities through its regulation of hormones secreted by the hypothalamus, pituitary, and adrenal glands. The hypothalamus and pituitary glands are located in the brain and are involved in mood regulation, while the adrenal glands sit atop the kidneys and help address stress in the body. The researchers concluded that frankincense has potential as a novel treatment for depression.

LAVENDER
(*Lavandula angustifolia*)

Lavender use has been traced back at least 2,500 years, when it was used for mummification and perfumery by the ancient Egyptians, Phoenicians, and Arabs. Today, science is revealing lavender's incredible ability to help reduce depression, premenstrual syndrome (PMS), and anxiety, as well as combating insomnia and repelling insects. A joint Canadian and Iranian study compared the effects of a medication for depression to drinking tea made from lavender flowers. The study found that lavender was about as effective as a common drug used in the treatment of depression. While the study was conducted using the flowers, lavender essential oil, which is extracted from lavender flowers, would likely have the same effect. Another study found that inhaling the scent of lavender essential oil every eight hours for four weeks immediately following pregnancy can significantly reduce the risk of postpartum depression, which can be serious and long-lasting in many women.

LEMON
(*Citrus limon*)

The fresh, bright scent of lemon is valuable for more than just cleaning your home; it can help ward off depression. According to a study in the journal *Behavioural Brain Research*, scientists found that lemon has antidepressant-like effects and is effective in the treatment of depression.

ORANGE
(*Citrus sinensis*)

In a study published in the medical journal *Physiology & Behavior*, researchers divided study participants in a dental office into two groups: those who were subjected to orange essential oil prior to dental treatments and those who were not subjected to the smell of any oil before their dental appointments. People were evaluated and those who inhaled orange oil prior to their treatment had lower levels of anxiety, increased calmness, and a better mood than the others.

ROSEMARY
(*Rosmarinus officinalis*)

Rosemary essential oil has been found to have a potent antidepressant effect on animals studied. Researchers found that the long-term traditional use of rosemary as a treatment for depression was justified. In the study, published in the *Journal of Ethnopharmacology*, the essential oil reversed depression about as well as the antidepressant drug fluoxetine.

You can diffuse one or more of the above essential oils in an essential oil diffuser to reap their antidepressant effects, or you simply inhale the oil several times throughout the day for at least a few minutes each time. Alternatively, carry a cloth to which you add a few drops of the oil and sniff it throughout the day, or place the cloth on your pillow to breathe in the scent while you sleep.

MOOD MAGIC CAPSULES

If you're suffering from depression, this blend of powerful antidepressant essential oils may be helpful, but you'll need to use them on a regular and consistent basis for best results.

Yield: 1 dose

* 1 drop bergamot essential oil
* 1 drop frankincense essential oil
* 1 drop lemon essential oil
* 1 drop wild orange essential oil
* 1 empty capsule
* Olive oil (optional)

Add the essential oils to an empty capsule and replace capsule top. If you have an irritable stomach, top up with a small amount of olive oil. Start with one capsule daily with food for a week and then move up to two capsules daily for another week, before increasing to, and sticking with, three capsules daily with meals, for at least one month.

DOWN-WITH-DEPRESSION ROLLERBALL

Keep this convenient rollerball handy to use throughout the day to help you deal with stress and to uplift your spirits.

Yield: 1 (10-milliliter) bottle

* 10 drops bergamot essential oil
* 10 drops lavender essential oil
* 10 drops wild orange essential oil
* Fractionated coconut oil or other carrier oil

Add the essential oils to an empty 10-milliliter rollerball bottle. Top up with fractionated coconut oil. Replace the rollerball top and cap. Shake gently to combine. Apply on the insides of your wrists and back of your neck three times daily for at least one month.

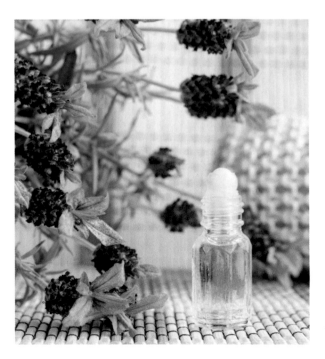

WORRY-FREE MIND DIFFUSER BLEND

Diffuse this blend when you need a mood boost, to alleviate worries and stresses, and to help deal with depression or anxiety.

Yield: 1 use

- ✳ 3 drops bergamot essential oil
- ✳ 2 drops lavender essential oil
- ✳ 2 drops wild orange essential oil

Add the essential oils to a diffuser. Diffuse for twenty minutes, three times daily, for at least a month.

TRANSFORMED OUTLOOK DIFFUSER BLEND

This diffuser blend, when used regularly, can help pull you out of darkness to have a more light-filled outlook.

Yield: 1 use

- ✳ 2 drops frankincense essential oil
- ✳ 2 drops rosemary essential oil
- ✳ 3 drops wild orange essential oil

Add the essential oils to a diffuser. Diffuse for twenty minutes, three times daily, for at least a month.

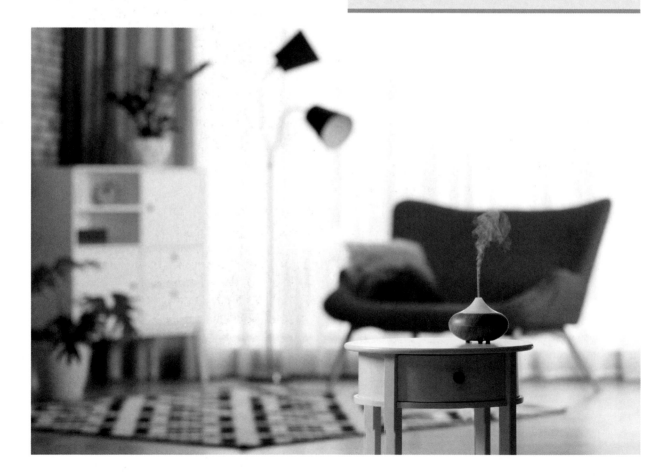

Essential Oils to Soothe Anxiety

If you suffer from an anxiety disorder or occasionally experience panic attacks, you might want to consider these four essential oils, all of which have proven anti-anxiety properties, without the side effects of anti-anxiety drugs.

BERGAMOT
(Citrus bergamia)

One study showed that bergamot essential oil quickly and effectively improved feelings of anxiety. In another study published in the medical journal *Phytotherapy Research,* scientists found that inhaling the essential oil of bergamot had a pronounced anti-anxiety effect. Excessively high levels of stress hormones are contributing factors in anxiety. According to their research, bergamot seemed to work by reducing the body's stress hormone production.

LAVENDER
(Lavandula angustifolia)

In a study published in the *Journal of Ethnopharmacology,* researchers found that animals that breathed the scent of lavender essential oil had significantly less anxiety. There are no known negative side effects of smelling lavender essential oil on a regular basis. Compare that to diazepam, which can leave you with blurred vision, drowsiness, constipation, dizziness, fatigue, headaches, mood problems, memory loss, hallucinations, slurred speech, trouble walking, trouble urinating, disinterest in sex, tremors, and sleep disturbances.

ROSE
(Rosa damascena)

In a study published in the journal *Pharmacology, Biochemistry, & Behavior,* researchers found that rose essential oil was effective for reducing feelings of conflict linked to anxiety. That's good news for anxiety sufferers interested in alternatives to the drugs and their many side effects.

VETIVER
(Chrysopogon zizanioides)

Research in the medical journal *Natural Product Research* also explored the effects of vetiver essential oil compared to the drug diazepam in its ability to reduce anxiety. Inhalation of vetiver essential oil had a comparable effect to the anti-anxiety drug. However, like lavender, vetiver has not been linked to the many side effects of diazepam and offers other health benefits like relaxation and improved sleep.

There are different ways to obtain the anti-anxiety benefits of these essential oils. You can add the oils to a handkerchief and breathe in the scent throughout the day, or use a diffuser or nebulizer. Heat can chemically alter the oils so it is preferable to choose options that do not involve heating them. Nebulizers are devices that spray microscopic particles of essential oils into the air. Either type of device can be found in many health food stores.

Eliminate Nutrient Deficiencies: Because so many vitamins and minerals are involved with mood balancing, it is important that you address any possible deficiencies by taking a high-quality multivitamin and mineral supplement with meals.

Boost Mood with B Vitamins: Because the B-complex vitamins are vital for brain health and balancing moods, a 100-milligram B-complex supplement daily is often necessary for people suffering from depression or brain neurotransmitter imbalances.

Provide the Precursor to Serotonin: A precursor to serotonin, 5-HTP helpt to restore healthy levels of this much needed brain chemical. I usually recommend people with depression use 50 to 100 milligrams of 5-HTP at bedtime for two months.

Regulate Brain Chemistry with SAMe: S-Adenosylmethionine (SAMe) occurs naturally in the body and helps regulate certain biochemical reactions, including those linked to mood regulation; however, it can be low in people suffering from anxiety or depression. Supplement with 400 to 1,600 milligrams daily of SAMe to ensure your brain can make important mood-elevating hormones.

Get the Sunshine Vitamin: Getting enough vitamin D on a daily basis can help with anxiety and depression, because it helps the body make serotonin. The best way to do that is through moderate sun exposure and vitamin D_3 supplementation.

Exercise Your Way to Brain Health: People suffering from imbalanced brain hormones should also supplement their daily routines through more fresh air and physical activity. Exercise is a natural antidepressant and anxiolytic (something that alleviates anxiety), and engaging in regular cardiovascular exercise like brisk walking or jogging is good for your body, mind, and spirit.

Rehydrate to Ensure Healthy Brain Signals: Did you know that your brain is electrical? It conducts electricity as a means of communication. And guess what helps to ensure the brain signals reach each other intact? Water. Without adequate water, brain neurotransmitters can't form properly or communicate effectively, so it is important to stay hydrated every day.

Ditching Perfume and Other Scented Products for Better Brain Health

Before you take a chance on Chanel's Chance or seek Amazing Grace (the perfume), you might want to rethink your decision to spritz yourself or your clothes. That's because most perfumes are made from toxic, synthetic ingredients that can destroy your hormonal health, brain health, and overall health. While humans have worn natural essential oils of herbs, flowers, and other natural substances for thousands of years, in recent decades, manufacturers of perfumes have switched to cheaper and increasingly toxic ingredients that are linked with a whole host of health problems. These ingredients can also be found in the perfumes that are added to laundry detergent, fabric softeners, and room "deodorizers." And don't forget

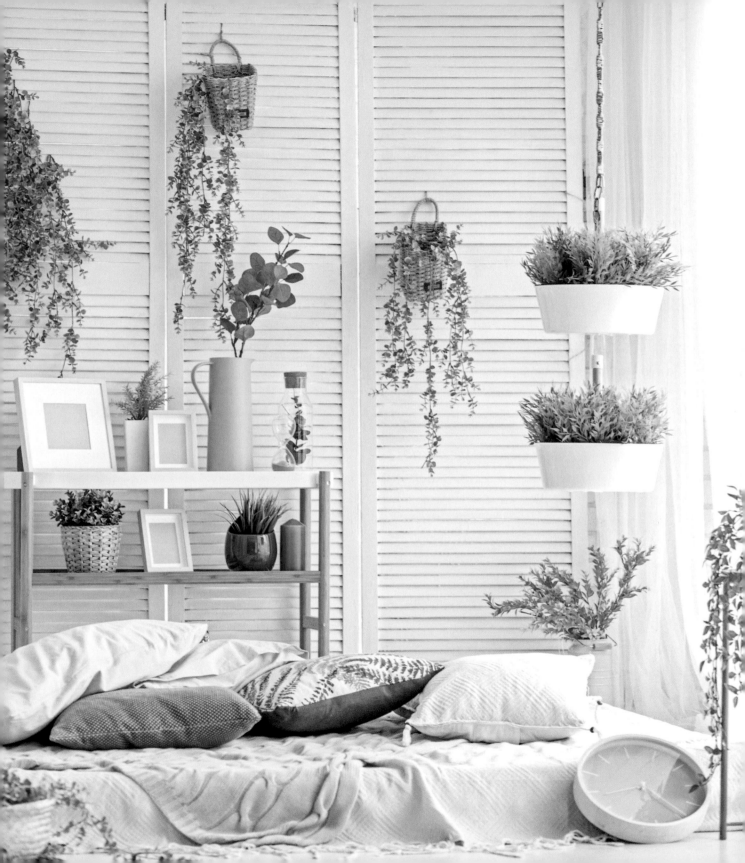

scented candles, as they contain many of the same nasty, potentially health-damaging ingredients.

What can you expect if you ditch perfume? You'll be amazed at how much better you'll feel. It may not happen overnight as it can take time to undo any preexisting damage you've experienced from using perfumes and colognes and for these toxic substances to be eliminated from your body and for your body to repair any damage. So, be patient. Most people notice improvements within a month of eliminating perfumes and colognes.

I can personally attest that I experienced most of the following health benefits and noticed that my sense of smell significantly improved. My husband jokingly says I have the sense of smell of a bloodhound, with an ability to smell things that seem to go unnoticed by most people. I also noticed my moods significantly improved. Years ago, I observed that after walking through the perfume counter at a department store, I would frequently come home exhausted and start to feel depressed. Once I avoided those stores and stopped using perfumes altogether, I experienced improved energy and fewer feelings of depression.

Most of my clients were shocked at how much better they feel after eliminating perfumes, colognes, scented laundry soap, fabric softeners, and other artificially-scented products from their daily life. And, most of them reported that when they stopped using their favorite perfume for a while and then smelled it again, they could not believe that they once loved it. It now smelled disgusting to them.

If you're dealing with any health issues, including anxiety or depression, I urge you to ditch perfumes, colognes, scented laundry products, fabric softeners, and other scented household and personal care products, as they can interfere with brain and other hormones. It's easier than you think.

Here are some of the many health benefits of purging artificial perfumes based on information from the chemical industry's own safety data sheets and the Environmental Health Network's findings regarding the most common chemicals found in the most popular perfumes.

Fewer Headaches: Chemicals like benzyl alcohol and methylene chloride are known to cause headaches.

Improved Moods: The methylene chloride used in perfume can cause irritability.

Reduced Incidence of Depression or Anxiety: The ethanol and linalool in many perfumes are known to disrupt the central nervous system, which may be linked to feelings of depression or anxiety.

Reduced Risk of Brain Disease: Some perfume chemicals have been linked to attention deficit disorder (ADD), Alzheimer's disease, dementia, multiple sclerosis, and Parkinson's disease. Acetone and benzyl alcohol specifically are linked to disturbances in the central nervous system.

Better Breathing: Benzaldehyde, benzyl acetate, ethanol, ethyl acetate, and linalool, commonly found in most perfumes, have all been linked to respiratory irritation and disturbances.

Improved Muscle Coordination: Benzyl alcohol and ethanol are known to cause muscle twitching and lack of coordination.

Improved Sense of Smell: Most of my clients report an improved sense of smell after eliminating perfumes. While I haven't seen the research on it, I believe that one or more chemicals in perfumes may impair it.

Less Pain: Many chemicals in perfumes are linked to pain. Benzyl aldehyde is linked to abdominal pain, while benzyl alcohol and methylene chloride are linked to headache pain.

Less Risk of Kidney or Liver Damage: The ethyl acetate used in many perfumes has been linked to both kidney and liver damage.

Reduced Risk of Cancer: Many perfumes contain many cancer-causing ingredients, including benzyl acetate, limonene, and methylene chloride. Benzyl acetate has been linked to one of the most deadly forms of cancer—pancreatic cancer.

BETTER-THAN-PERFUME ROLLERBALL BLEND

Skip the toxic, brain-damaging perfumes on the market that are mostly derived from petrochemicals. Use this brain-uplifting blend as a natural perfume instead.

Yield: 1 (10-milliliter) bottle

* 5 drops lavender essential oil
* 5 drops rose essential oil
* 10 drops ylang-ylang essential oil
* Fractionated coconut oil or other carrier oil

Add the essential oils to an empty 10-milliliter rollerball bottle. Top up with fractionated coconut oil. Replace the rollerball top and cap. Gently shake until combined. Apply on the inside of your wrists and on your neck, as desired.

BETTER-THAN-COLOGNE ROLLERBALL BLEND

This blend of woodsy essential oils is far superior to the commercially-available ones derived from petrochemicals, and actually boosts your brain and adrenal gland health at the same time.

Yield: 1 (10-milliliter) bottle

* 10 drops Siberian fir essential oil
* 3 drops cedar essential oil
* 5 drops black spruce essential oil
* Fractionated coconut oil or other carrier oil

Add the essential oils to an empty 10-milliliter rollerball bottle. Top up with fractionated coconut oil. Replace the rollerball top and cap. Gently shake until combined. Apply on the inside of your wrists and on your neck, as desired.

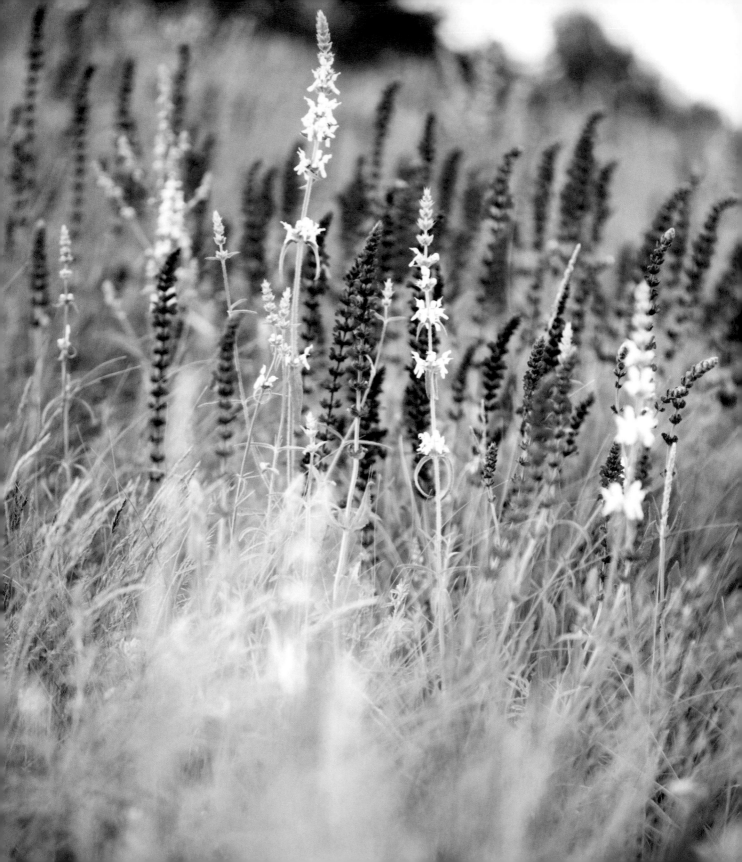

6

Ovary Renewal
The Hormones of Womanhood

THE PATH FROM GIRLHOOD TO WOMANHOOD, through middle-age and eventually into the wise woman years, is typically filled with many joys and challenges along the way. Regardless of the phase you are currently experiencing, you can be assured that hormones are playing a critical role in your health and feelings of joy. They determine when you start menstruating, how frequently, and how difficult it may be. They determine, at least in part, whether we have children, how soon we will live independently of our monthly cycles, and how painful or painless all of these events may be. They determine our sex drive or lack thereof, and even play a role in how pleasurable sex may be.

Society often treats the various phases of womanhood as disease states, and sadly, many health practitioners treat women's health as nothing more than an inconvenience. The reality could not be further from the truth. Womanhood is a powerful combination of strength and gentility, intelligence and wisdom. This approach to women and their health shows an inherent bias and misunderstanding, and frankly, a lack of respect for the beautiful and powerful woman's body—the place from which all human life and great amounts of joy originate.

Many people in our Western culture continue to denigrate "that time of the month," call the weight gain during the midlife as "menopot," or use some other derogatory expression to describe our femaleness, but menstruation and menopause are not illnesses. We need to view womanhood from a position of strength and power and not one of victimhood. Our hormonal fluctuations and differing phases of our lives give us a unique ability to purify our body, increase our connection with our inner knowing and nature, and boost our strength and power as women. We are inherently powerful beings.

While it may feel difficult to celebrate these milestones when you are suffering through them in ill health and with hormonal imbalances, essential oils can help you to rebalance your hormones and gain a healthy relationship with your body, heal any wounds you may be carrying, and reconnect with your natural female strength and power. They can make it possible to enjoy whatever stage of life you are in, free from imbalanced hormones and the difficult symptoms that can result.

As we explore the various hormonally linked stages of womanhood, including menstruation and fertility, the transitional years of perimenopause, the freedom of menopause, and the wise woman years, it is my hope that you will embrace the beauty and wisdom available to you during these phases. During our discussion of each stage, I'll share some of the best remedies to address the symptoms of hormonal imbalance so you can better embrace the stage of life you're in.

The Powerful Female Hormonal System

The female endocrine system contains the ovaries, which are responsible for the production of eggs and for the secretion of hormones like estrogen and progesterone. I'll explain more about these hormones momentarily, but for now, it is important to know that these hormones play integral roles in a woman's reproductive, emotional, and physical health. Estrogen and progesterone regulate countless functions in a woman's body. Estrogen, for example, helps to regulate mood, sleep, energy levels, bone density, memory, and sex drive. Progesterone helps to regulate skin health, fertility, blood circulation, and even whether you'll suffer from varicose veins or heart palpitations. Together, they influence energy levels and happiness, and ensure healthy bones. Within seconds of their production in the ovaries, the blood transports these hormones anywhere they need to go in the body.

Menstruation and Fertility

Menstruation represents an opportunity that is exclusively available to women—to reproduce, or not, as we desire. It is also an opportunity that the body takes on a monthly basis to cleanse itself of harmful toxins and emotions that may be holding us back from achieving our full potential.

Sadly, as is often the case for many young women, the transition from girlhood to womanhood often arrives not with fanfare but with the jarring thud of painful abdominal cramping, anxiety, depression, fatigue, headaches or migraines, skin breakouts, bloating, and unhealthy food cravings. For some women, symptoms such as cramps can be mild while others experience debilitating pain that can affect their ability to work, attend school, and participate in athletics or social activities. Dysmenorrhea—the medical term for painful periods—seriously affects at least sixty percent of women and their quality of life.

These symptoms frequently accompany a woman's periods throughout her life and can signal that our bodies are experiencing some degree of hormonal imbalance, but this suffering is largely unnecessary, particularly when there are so many powerful, natural herb-based medicines that can restore our sense of well-being and alleviate any discomfort we may be experiencing.

Most women's monthly cycles range between 26 and 35 days. The cycle is maintained through the secretion of, as well as the ebb and flow of, sex hormones. They maintain this cycle and regulate when you get your periods, how short or long they will last, how heavy or light they will be, and whether they will be regular.

During menstruation, the hormones estrogen and progesterone, among others, rise and fall to prepare a woman's body for a possible pregnancy. Typically, estrogen rises during the first half of a woman's monthly cycle and drops in the second half. For women with PMS, the brain hormone serotonin also frequently drops alongside the lower estrogen levels, which can create a recipe for cramps, depression, and other undesirable symptoms. (Learn more about how to boost serotonin levels in chapter 5, page 101.) Low levels of the hormone progesterone may result in a shorter-than-average monthly cycle (less than 26 days).

Do You Suffer from Premenstrual Syndrome (PMS)?

While various experts state that PMS affects between eight and fifteen percent of women during their reproductive years, I believe that number may actually be much higher since most women never report their symptoms to a doctor. Premenstrual syndrome, also known as premenstrual tension (PMT), can cause a wide range of symptoms, including breast tenderness, depression, anxiety, abdominal bloating, appetite changes, insomnia, and many others. While many thoughtless people (typically those who have never experienced just how severe PMS can be) make the condition the topic of jokes, the sad reality for many women is that PMS can be excruciatingly painful and even destructive to quality of life and the ability to work. When premenstrual syndrome is that severe and even debilitating, it is given the medical diagnosis of premenstrual dysphoric disorder (PMDD).

SUCCESS STORY:
Barbara Beats Hot Flashes

discovered how powerful medical aroma-therapy can be many years ago thanks to Barbara, a woman in her early fifties who worked as an administrator of a large orga-nization, who experienced horrible hot flashes that robbed her of sleep. She never slept for more than two hours at a time before waking up in a pool of sweat. This happened daily and left her feeling com-pletely exhausted and unable to function. She had tried the pharmaceutical drugs prescribed to her without improvement. She had also visited many naturally minded practitioners and tried the commonly rec-ommended black cohosh and other herbs and supplements typically given to women suffering from hot flashes.

Since her suffering was so severe and her improvement nonexistent, I knew she needed something more powerful. Normally, some dietary changes, a couple of nutrients, and an herbal remedy would have most of my menopausal clients singing, but Barbara didn't respond to any of the standard nat-ural treatments.

I started lesser-known options like the medical use of essential oils. So, I gave her my Menopause Magic Rollerball Blend (page 136)—an essential oil blend to help balance her hormones—which I instructed her to apply to her inner wrists, neck, and abdomen, at least three times daily and to deeply inhale the aroma for at least a couple of minutes each time she applied it. Et voila! Her symptoms were almost completely gone within several days. We were both ecstatic. Since then, when noth-ing else seems to work, I bring out the "big guns"—the delicate oils of flowers, seeds, and leaves.

She called a week later to tell me that her hot flashes were nearly gone. When she returned for her monthly check-up, she was free of them completely after they had plagued her for years. Her eyes welled up with tears as she described the improve-ment and how she finally felt like she was back to her vibrant self.

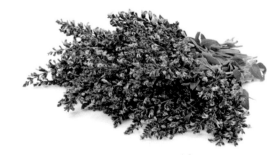

Essential Oils to Nix PMS Symptoms

Regardless whether you suffer from PMS or PMDD, you'll be happy to know that you can use many of the essential oils and remedies described throughout this chapter to address their symptoms. Even women who declared that they had "tried everything" were astounded at how effective the correct application of the best essential oils, taken in the ideal dose, transformed their life. Essential oils combined with a low-sugar, reduced-meat, and increased plant-based diet can alleviate symptoms (see 10-Day Plan, page 44).

LAVENDER
(Lavandula angustifolia)

For women suffering from premenstrual syndrome, research shows that lavender is helpful for reducing emotional issues attributed to monthly hormonal fluctuations. A new study published in the journal *BioPsychoSocial Medicine* found that inhaling the scent of lavender for 10 minutes had a significant effect on the nervous system of women suffering from premenstrual symptoms. It especially decreased feelings of depression and confusion linked to PMS. To alleviate mood-related PMS symptoms, place a few drops of lavender essential oil on a handkerchief and inhale periodically, make a tea from dried flowers, or regularly breathe deeply of a plant growing indoors or outdoors.

FENNEL
(Foeniculum vulgare)

The seeds and extracts made from the fennel seeds have science-proven abilities to improve digestion, reduce symptoms linked to menstruation, and act as an anti-spasmodic.

In an animal study published in the *Journal of Ethnopharmacology*, researchers found that fennel essential oil was effective at reducing the intensity and frequency of menstrual abdominal contractions linked to inflammatory compounds known as prostaglandins.

Another study published in the *Iranian Journal of Nursing and Midwifery Research* assessed the effectiveness of fennel, along with vitamin E, in comparison to ibuprofen. While both the fennel and ibuprofen showed effectiveness against pain, the fennel demonstrated greater effectiveness, particularly after 1–2 hours after administration and its overall ability to alleviate pain was superior to the ibuprofen, which can have side effects including nausea, dyspepsia, diarrhea, and fatigue, and has been linked to liver damage.

The scientists who conducted this study believe its analgesic effect may be largely due to fennel's anethole content, since this ingredient is best known for its anti-spasmodic actions. Additionally, anethole joins to the body's dopamine receptors to decrease pain.

While the study used an alcohol extract of the herb, oil extracts of fennel also contain anethole, making the use of fennel essential oil a good way to reap the benefits of the herb. Apply diluted fennel essential oil over the abdominal area a few times daily, not just during periods but throughout the month. If the product you select can be used internally, you can also take one drop of fennel essential oil on your tongue or in a glass of water or juice three times daily throughout the month to reduce cramps when you get your period.

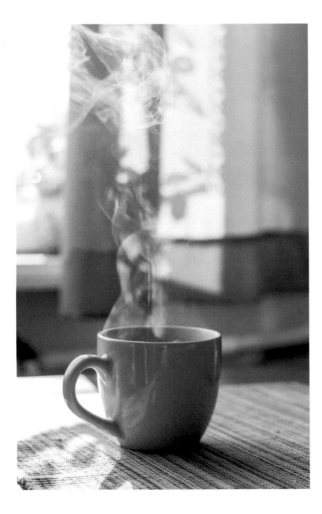

PMS BE GONE BLEND

While many women suffer through PMS symptoms or pop over-the-counter drugs, regularly inhaling certain essential oils like clary sage can minimize PMS symptoms or eliminate them altogether.

Yield: 1 application

* 1 drop clary sage essential oil
* 5 drops fractionated coconut oil

Put the drop of clary sage oil in the 5 drops of coconut oil. Apply a drop of the blend to the inside of your wrists, three times daily, for at least a month, to help balance hormones and alleviate PMS.

PMS TAMER DIFFUSER BLEND

This anti-PMS blend incorporates four powerful oils that, on their own, are helpful for PMS. When combined and used regularly, they work like magic.

Yield: 1 use

* 3 drops clary sage essential oil
* 2 drops lavender essential oil
* 1 drop peppermint essential oil
* 2 drops ylang-ylang essential oil

Add the essential oils to a diffuser and run for twenty minutes, three times daily, throughout the month, especially during your menstrual cycle.

DR. COOK'S CRAMP BUSTER

Menstrual cramps typically start before or with menstrual flow, and are frequently accompanied by nausea, vomiting, headaches, and faintness. Every woman who has ever experienced painful menstrual cramps knows the importance of pain relief. The following blend can help.

Yield: 1 (10-milliliter) bottle

* 10 drops clary sage essential oil
* 10 drops copaiba essential oil
* 10 drops fennel essential oil
* 3 drops lavender essential oil
* 2 drops rosemary essential oil
* Fractionated coconut oil or other carrier oil

In an empty 10-milliliter rollerball bottle, add the essential oils. Top up the bottle with fractionated coconut oil. Replace the rollerball top and cap and gently shake until well combined. Apply to your abdomen at the first sign of cramps and repeat as necessary, up to five times daily.

CRAMPS BE GONE ROLLERBALL

Don't just suffer with cramps. Keep this convenient rollerball bottle of oils handy, and regularly rub over your abdomen to alleviate cramps.

Yield: 1 (10-milliliter) bottle

* 15 drops clary sage essential oil
* 15 drops copaiba essential oil
* 5 drops geranium essential oil
* Fractionated coconut oil or other carrier oil

In an empty 10-milliliter rollerball bottle, add the essential oils. Top up with fractionated coconut or olive oil. Gently shake until combined. Roll over abdominal area as needed for relief of menstrual cramps.

Looking for More Help?

* If you experience PMS, you may feel depressed during the week before your period. There are mood-boosting essential oils that can help. See page 123 to learn more.

Honoring Your Feelings During Your Periods

Many years ago, I had a conversation with a colleague, who was a practicing psychologist. She felt that women needed to stop denigrating their feelings of irritability, sadness, or anger during their monthly periods and, instead, recognize that they may actually be the body's way for women to stop suppressing their true feelings as many women do throughout the rest of the month. She believed that, in our society, women are often shamed for feeling anger or irritation, particularly toward their partner. As a result, they often suppress these emotions until their monthly periods arrive and they can no longer keep them under wraps.

Regardless of whether you agree, there is value in recognizing and honoring your feelings and living a life of honesty with yourself about how you truly feel. In addition to working on the physical level of our being, essential oils can also help us to connect with our emotions and heal any emotional wounds we may be carrying, and fully own our strength.

Essential oils work for emotional healing on many levels. The simple art of making time for your healing can help to put you in touch with your feelings. The oils can help regulate brain neurotransmitters, which are closely linked to emotions. And each of the oils has an "emotional signature" in that it has certain emotional healing effects. For example, bergamot essential oil can help to alleviate feelings that we are unlovable, while black pepper essential oil has been used to encourage honesty with ourselves about how we are feeling. Spruce essential oil can help us feel more connected to others and the world in which we live.

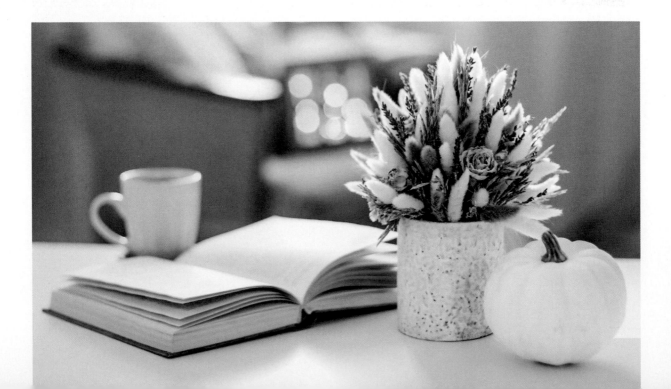

Essential Oils to Relieve Headaches and Migraines

Many women experience headaches or migraines either just before or during their periods. They are usually linked to the effects of sudden drops or increases in certain hormones. Regardless of whether you suffer from headaches or their much worse counterpart, migraines, essential oils can help.

Essential oils are powerful natural medicines that truly shine when it comes to addressing headaches. They quickly and effectively travel to the brain, inducing hormonal changes there or in the glands controlled by the brain. This means that they can get to the root of the problem for many women during their monthly cycles—the hormonal imbalances that can cause headaches or migraines. And, unlike many headache medications that are replete with horrible side effects, including liver damage, essential oils are much safer. Here are some of my top picks for headaches:

COPAIBA
(Copaifera reticulata, C. officinalis, C. coriacea, and C. langsdorffii)

One of the most potent anti-pain remedies available, copaiba has astounded everyone to whom I've ever recommended it with its quick and highly effective results. In addition to having the anti-inflammatory properties described in chapter 2, the BCP in copaiba works on the body's endocannabinoid system, which is a little-known but powerful system that controls pain, brain functions, immunity, and many hormones. BCP does not have psychoactive effects (unlike some of the cannabinoids in marijuana). In other words, it will help with pain without making you high. It can be used directly on the temples, back of the neck, or other places involved in headaches. I also use it internally for headaches or migraines, using three drops about three times a day.

EUCALYPTUS
(Eucalyptus globulus)

If your headaches are linked to sinus congestion, sinusitis, or a cold that involves sinus pressure, you'll want to try eucalyptus. Eucalyptus essential oil works to clear the sinuses, thereby relieving the pressure that's causing the headache. A few drops can be diluted in a carrier oil and applied to the chest. It can be used straight, which is known as "neat" in aromatherapy, in a diffuser. I find adding a few drops to a tissue or handkerchief and leaving it on my pillow before sleeping quickly alleviates sinus pressure and the headaches linked to it. Do not use internally.

LAVENDER
(Lavandula angustifolia)

Highly effective at reducing tension and stress, lavender is a great choice for headaches or migraines. Lavender essential oil has been found in a study published in the medical journal *European Neurology* to be a safe and effective treatment for alleviating migraines. Whether you're suffering from an occasional headache or debilitated by migraines, lavender, particularly combined with copaiba, is a great choice. Rub lavender oil on your neck, head, and forehead as well as diffuse it in a diffuser.

MARJORAM
(Origanum majorana)

If your headaches are linked to stress and tension, marjoram is an excellent choice to apply directly to the neck and shoulders, since tight muscles in these areas can often cause headaches. I find the combination of marjoram, copaiba, and peppermint particularly effective for this purpose.

PEPPERMINT
(Mentha piperita)

Peppermint essential oil is one of my favorite headache remedies of all time, and I have sent many clients home with a bottle to roll on or apply directly to their temples, or sore spots on their forehead, head, and back of the neck, particularly where the head meets the neck. Be careful not to use too much or the fumes will cause your eyes to water. Avoid getting the oil in your eyes and be sure to wash your hands immediately after use to prevent rubbing the peppermint oil into your eyes.

ROSE
(Rosa damascena)

Research in the medical journal *Complementary Therapies in Medicine* found that rose essential oil applied to sore areas of the head and neck may be helpful in the treatment and management of migraine headaches. It is an expensive oil but worth every penny as it offers profound healing, particularly when used alongside copaiba essential oil. If the rose essential oil you select is inexpensive, it is almost guaranteed to be diluted or cut with cheap or synthetic oils that are of no value. You really do get what you pay for when it comes to essential oils, especially rose oil.

In my many years of experience, I have found that topical and ingestion of one or more of the above oils tend to yield the best results for headaches. However, not all oils are suitable for ingestion. Most are not. Remember, use only oils that clearly indicate their suitability for internal use. Oils like copaiba and peppermint tend to be good choices for this purpose.

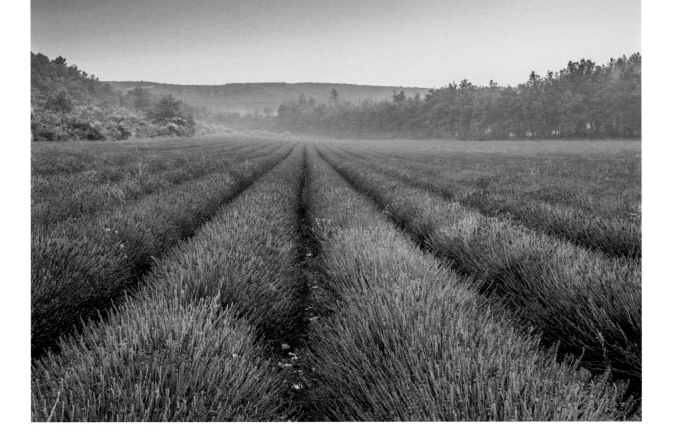

MIGRAINE MAGIC ROLLERBALL

This blend of oils can help reduce the nasty pain of migraine headaches.

Yield: 1 (10-milliliter) bottle

- * 40 drops copaiba essential oil
- * 40 drops peppermint essential oil
- * Fractionated coconut oil or other carrier oil

Add the essential oils to a 10-milliliter empty rollerball bottle. Top up the bottle with fractionated coconut oil. Replace the rollerball and cap. Gently shake until the oils are mixed. Apply to the inner wrists or neck whenever you're feeling migraine pain.

MIGRAINE MIRACLE

Ideally, use this migraine formula at the same time as using the Migraine Magic Rollerball, since the combination of topical use of the latter formula combined with internal use of this one addresses migraines on multiple levels.

Yield: Approximately 10 milliliters

- * 50 drops copaiba essential oil
- * 50 drops peppermint essential oil

In a small bottle, combine the copaiba and peppermint essential oils. Gently shake until well mixed. Take four drops on your tongue when you feel a migraine starting. Take an additional four drops every hour or two to a maximum of twenty drops of all oils combined on any given day.

Pregnancy and Labor

The use of essential oils during pregnancy or breastfeeding is slightly controversial. Physicians are often cautious to recommend anything during these times to avoid any possible harm to an unborn or developing baby. As a result, most aromatherapists tend to avoid recommending any essential oils at least during the first trimester of pregnancy, and others don't recommend them at all during these periods.

Much of the concern may be unfounded; however, there are few studies of the effects of essential oils during pregnancy or breastfeeding, making it difficult to know for sure if there is any potential danger.

One study conducted by Ethel Burns and her team at Oxford University assessed the effects of clary sage, eucalyptus (globulus), frankincense, jasmine, lavender, lemon, mandarin, peppermint, Roman chamomile, and rose during labor. She collected evidence on 8,058 women in labor and published her findings showing the effectiveness of the blend. However, it is best to proceed with caution and consult a doctor (see page 4 for additional guidelines).

DR. COOK'S FERTILITY BLEND

This blend contains several excellent oils that help balance hormones and promote fertility.

Yield: 1 (10-milliliter) bottle

* 10 drops bergamot essential oil
* 15 drops clary sage essential oil
* 12 drops fennel essential oil
* 10 drops geranium essential oil
* 10 drops lavender essential oil
* Fractionated coconut oil or other carrier oil

Place the oils in an empty 10-milliliter rollerball bottle. Top up with fractionated coconut oil. Apply to the abdomen and inside of wrists twice daily. Inhale deeply each time.

DR. COOK'S ANTI–STRETCH MARK BLEND

You can use the following blend after the first trimester of pregnancy, throughout the remainder of your pregnancy, or afterward if you already have stretch marks from previous pregnancies.

Yield: 1 (10-milliliter) bottle

* 30 drops mandarin essential oil
* 30 drops rose hip seed oil
* Fractionated coconut oil

Place the oils in an empty 10-milliliter rollerball bottle. Top up with fractionated coconut oil. Apply to abdomen and other places you may have stretch marks at least once a day on an ongoing basis.

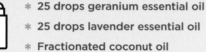
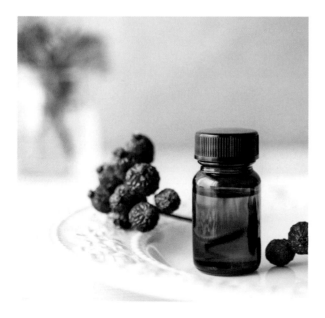

The Wise Woman Years

While our society tends to place an unhealthy focus on youth, I noticed in my practice that many women become stronger and more confident in their midlife years and afterward. It is time to celebrate this powerful phase of a woman's life as a true coming-in-to-her-own. Reducing any uncomfortable hormonal symptoms you may be experiencing as your body adjusts to the transition will help you fully honor your strength as a woman.

Perimenopause

Are you suffering from a range of unexpected and undesired symptoms that have left you scratching your head in confusion? You may be experiencing the perimenopause—a woman's natural transition between her potentially childbearing years and menopause, which usually lasts two to ten years, depending on the woman. Technically, perimenopause is the time of a woman's life when she starts experiencing menstrual changes up to ten years prior to menopause. Most women start experiencing perimenopause in their forties, but some women start as early as their mid-thirties. While it is a natural and normal experience in a woman's life, that doesn't mean it is always easy. Some women may have no symptoms at all; other women suffer from a whole range of uncomfortable to downright difficult symptoms.

Here are some of the most common symptoms that may be experienced during perimenopause:

* Abdominal fat increases
* Anemia (if your periods become heavy)
* Anxiety

* Bone mass loss
* Depression
* Difficulty handling stress
* Fatigue
* Fibrocystic breasts
* Heavy periods
* Hot flashes
* Incontinence
* Increased cholesterol levels
* Irritability
* Menstrual changes
* Migraines
* Missed periods
* Mood swings
* Muscle loss
* Nausea
* Night sweats
* Painful or uncomfortable intercourse (thinning of vaginal tissues and vaginal dryness can make intercourse painful for some women)
* Reduced fertility (as long as you're experiencing periods, you're most likely ovulating, which means you may still be able to become pregnant)
* Reduced libido
* Scant or light periods
* Sleep disturbances
* Sore breasts

* Urinary tract infections (hormonal fluctuations may make you more vulnerable to urinary tract infections)
* Vaginal dryness
* Weight gain

Essential Oils for Perimenopause

Many of the essential oils that address estrogen and progesterone imbalances (you'll learn more about these conditions on pages 137 and 141) can help with the symptoms of perimenopause, but it is important to mention one oil in particular.

GERANIUM
(Pelargonium graveolens)

Geranium essential oil has been found to be helpful for healing emotions linked to imbalanced hormones during perimenopause. In a study published in the journal *Neuroendocrinology Letters*, researchers found that the essential oil's effectiveness may be linked to its ability to restore falling estrogen levels.

It's important to remember that it is natural to feel emotional during any transitional phase of life. Many women feel grief and sadness as they prepare to move out of having childbearing potential into the wise woman years.

PERIMENOPAUSAL EMOTIONAL HEALING MASSAGE BLEND

This massage blend doesn't just smell heavenly. It also helps to reset hormones linked to perimenopausal symptoms.

Yield: 1 (10-milliliter) bottle

* 20 drops geranium essential oil
* 8 drops lavender essential oil
* 2 drops rose essential oil (optional)
* Fractionated coconut oil or other carrier oil

Add the essential oils to an empty 10-milliliter rollerball bottle. Top up with fractionated coconut oil. Replace the rollerball and cap. Gently shake until the oils are mixed. Apply to the inner wrists or neck whenever you're feeling overwhelmed with sadness or grief.

Menopause

Menopause is the natural end of women's fertile years; it often brings great freedom for many women. It is a transformative time in a woman's life. While many women experience some degree of grief over the loss of the capacity to bear children, most are also thrilled with their newfound freedom from periods or pregnancy. In my natural medicine practice, I frequently observed women owning their strength and power, and transforming their lives during the menopausal years. It often amazed me how many would choose to end cycles of abuse, hone their artistic and literary talents, opt for a new career path, embark upon adventurous travels, or make other great life changes during menopause.

Menopause begins one year after the cessation of the last period, and while it typically occurs when a woman reaches her fifties, it can begin earlier than that for some women. During this time, the ovaries no longer release an egg for conception every month and stop producing significant amounts of estrogen and progesterone, causing changes in a woman's cycle and potentially some unwanted symptoms, which can include aching joints, brain fog, dry skin, depression, fatigue, hot flashes, heart palpitations, irritable bowel syndrome, lower libido, memory loss, mood swings, osteoporosis, nausea, sleep disorders, vaginal dryness, weight changes, as well as an increased risk of heart disease. That doesn't mean that heart disease is an inevitable effect of menopause; it simply means it is important to take dietary and lifestyle measures to reduce your risk.

Further research into certain oils, such as laurel leaf, clary sage, and peppermint, showed that they had estrogen-like properties, balanced the nervous system, and eased pain and spasms. The same blend of oils worked for women suffering from PMS, menopause, endometriosis, pelvic pain, painful periods, and more.

Essential Oils to Keep Handy During Menopause

Menopause can be one of the most freeing times in a woman's life, but if you're experiencing hot flashes, headaches, a waning libido, stress, or other unwanted symptoms, you may not be experiencing life to its fullest. To help you address any symptoms that may arise, I've compiled this list of essential oils to keep on hand. Of course, every woman's experiences during the menopausal years is different, so if you're experiencing other symptoms, don't forget to look them up throughout this book.

CLARY SAGE
(Salvia sclarea)

Clary sage is the perfect oil to keep on hand throughout the menopausal years. Sclareol found in clary sage helps to restore estrogen balance in women whose levels may have waned during menopause; inhalation or topical application may also help with hot flashes. You can use the PMS Be Gone Blend (see page 124), a combination of clary sage oil and coconut oil, to help balance hormones and alleviate menopausal symptoms.

COPAIBA
(Copaifera reticulata, C. officinalis, C. coriacea, and C. langsdorffii)

Many women suffer from pain or headaches during the menopausal years. Keep copaiba handy to apply topically to painful areas, or take a few drops on the tongue or in an empty capsule to help control pain.

GERANIUM
(Pelargonium graveolens)

Geranium essential oil may help restore balance to moods and lend emotional support during menopause. In a study published in the journal *Neuroendocrinology Letters*, researchers found that the essential oil's effectiveness may be linked to its ability to restore falling estrogen levels. It also helps to boost declining libido that frequently occurs in menopause.

JASMINE
(Jasminum grandiflorum)

A natural aphrodisiac, jasmine essential oil can help boost a waning libido which is common during menopause, and often helps to boost a woman's feelings of being desirable and sensual.

LAVENDER
(Lavandula angustifolia)

Many women experience trouble sleeping during the menopausal years, often due to hot flashes. Fortunately, lavender can help you address insomnia and to achieve a deeper, more restful night's sleep. Apply a drop or two on the soles of your feet or palms of your hands within an hour of retiring to bed or as needed during the night to help you sleep. Also place a drop in your hands whenever you may be experiencing anxiety for quick relief.

MARJORAM
(Origanum majorana)

Let's face it: any life change can create tension and stress, which can in turn cause tight and sore muscles. Diluted marjoram essential oil can be applied to the neck and shoulders or anywhere your muscles are tight and sore. Combine with some copaiba essential oil to ease any inflammation and pain in these areas.

PEPPERMINT
(Mentha piperita)

When applied topically, peppermint can help cool the body during hot flashes; when used on the back of the head, neck, and temples, it can ease headaches that some women suffer from during their menopausal years. Because it contains the potent compound viridifloral, it can help to restore estrogen levels in the body.

ROSE
(Rosa damascena)

An aphrodisiac, rose essential oil can restore a waning libido and improve sexual function in women whose sex drive has taken a nosedive. Stick with it though since it can take a couple of months for its full effects.

STAR ANISE
(Illicium verum)

Like clary sage and peppermint, star anise can help to boost estrogen levels to ensure healthy bones during and after the menopausal years. Diffuse star anise essential oil, which contains anethole, for maximum benefit.

VETIVER
(Vetiveria zizanioides)

If hot flashes, pain, or other symptoms are keeping you awake at night, or preventing you from getting a restful night's sleep, apply a drop of vetiver to the soles of your feet before bed or whenever you awaken during the night.

MENOPAUSE MAGIC ROLLERBALL BLEND

The following blend of essential oils helps to address hormonal imbalances commonly experienced and is convenient to use on a regular basis.

Yield: 1 (10-milliliter) bottle

* 6 drops laurel leaf essential oil
* 6 drops niaouli essential oil
* 6 drops star anise essential oil
* 6 drops peppermint essential oil
* 6 drops clary sage essential oil
* Fractionated coconut oil or other carrier oil

Add the essential oils to an empty 10-milliliter rollerball bottle. Top up with fractionated coconut oil. Replace the rollerball top and cap. Gently shake to combine all oils. Apply to inner wrists or neck and deeply inhale aroma at least three times daily. Continue use every day for at least thirty days for optimal results.

DR. COOK'S HOT FLASH BLEND

The following blend of essential oils has been a life-saver for many of my menopausal clients who suffer from hot flashes. It has been effective for even the worst hot flashes, when used a few times a day, every day.

Yield: 1 (10-milliliter) bottle

* 10 drops clary sage essential oil
* 5 drops fennel essential oil
* 7 drops geranium essential oil
* 3 drops lavender essential oil
* 2 drops rosewood essential oil
* 2 drops ylang-ylang essential oil
* Fractionated coconut oil or other carrier oil

Add the essential oils to an empty 10-milliliter rollerball bottle. Top up with fractionated coconut oil. Replace the rollerball top and cap. Gently shake to combine all oils. Apply to your inner wrists or neck and deeply inhale the aroma at least three times daily. Continue use every day for at least thirty days for optimal results.

Balancing Haywire Estrogen Levels

Did you know that there are estrogen receptors found in cells throughout your body, including your brain, breasts, bones, and belly? It's true. Estrogen is a powerful hormone that affects almost every aspect of a women's hormonal and overall health. It is imperative to have adequate estrogen levels.

Do You Have Low Estrogen Levels?

There are many symptoms of low estrogen levels, some of which include the following symptoms or conditions. Keep in mind that it is not necessary to have all of the symptoms to be experiencing low estrogen levels, and if you suspect that you are suffering from any health issues, it is best to consult your physician.

* Amenorrhea (cessation of periods but not menopausal)
* Depression or mood swings
* Difficulty falling or staying asleep
* Dry eyes or cataracts (in women)
* Dry skin
* Fatigue
* Hair loss
* Headaches or migraines
* Hot flashes
* Infertility
* Irritability
* Loss of bone density or osteoporosis
* Love handles or abdominal fat (in menopausal women)
* Low libido
* Menopause
* Painful intercourse
* Poor concentration or memory
* Postpartum depression (depression after childbirth, which is usually the result of a significant drop in estrogen levels)
* Premenstrual syndrome with these specific symptoms: depression; sugar, bread, or pasta cravings; or low blood sugar
* Sagging or thinning skin
* Shrinking or sagging breasts
* Urinary incontinence
* Vaginal dryness

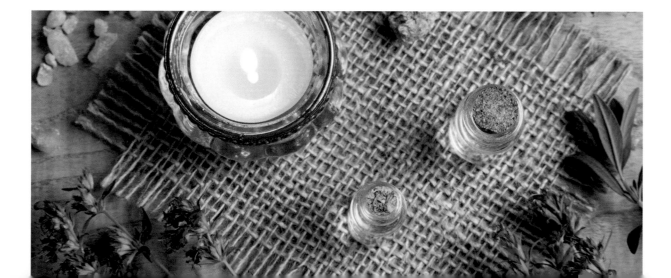

Essential Oils that Can Boost Estrogen Levels

There are many essential oils that can boost estrogen levels to help alleviate the symptoms of PMS, PDD, and menopausal symptoms. Some of the best ones include the following:

CLARY SAGE
(Salvia sclarea)

This go-to oil for female hormonal imbalances contains the compound known as sclareol, which regulates estrogen levels in the body. Because of its estrogen-like properties, clary sage essential oil can help balance hormones in menstruating, nursing, and menopausal women. It may decrease excessive menstruation and lactation and alleviate menopausal symptoms like hot flashes. Clary sage is also helpful for women whose periods have stopped or have not started, a condition known as amenorrhea. Inhalation of or massage with diluted clary sage essential oil is the most direct route of affecting hormones. If you're not sure which essential oil to use for women's health issues, grab clary sage. More often than not, it will help.

LEMONGRASS
(Cymbopogon flexuosus)

Lemongrass essential oil may be one of the best remedies to boost estrogen levels, especially for those who are suffering from the resulting PMS or menopausal symptoms that typically accompany low estrogen levels.

NIAOULI
(Melaleuca quinquenervia)

Niaouli contains the compound viridiflorol, which acts as an estrogen-like substance inside the body, helping to restore hormone levels.

PEPPERMINT
(Mentha piperita)

Peppermint is most known for its analgesic properties thanks to the naturally occurring substance known as menthol, but, like niaouli, it also contains viridifloral, which helps to restore estrogen levels in the body.

STAR ANISE
(Illicium verum)

With a delightful scent similar to licorice, pure star anise essential oil contains anethole, which helps to boost estrogen levels in those whose levels are low. Like clary sage, star anise is also beneficial for women whose periods have stopped but are not yet in their menopausal years.

Ideally, these oils can be made into a blend. While little research has been done on the effects of these essential oils on breast cancer, you may wish to avoid using them if you have the disease due to its sensitivity to estrogen.

Looking for More Help?

* A drop in estrogen, especially during menopause, can lead to hair loss or thinning hair. The oils on page 158 can help restore your tresses.

* To tackle mood-related symptoms related to low estrogen levels, harness the power of the mood-boosting oils recommended on page 107.

* If low estrogen levels have caused weight gain, the oils on page 89 can help boost your metabolism.

* For more info about boosting libido, see page 160.

DR. COOK'S BLEND FOR MISSING PERIODS

If you've stopped having periods and are not yet in your perimenopausal or menopausal years, you may want to use the following blend. The oils used here can help to activate periods when they have mysteriously stopped.

Yield: 1 (10-milliliter) bottle

* 20 drops geranium essential oil
* 10 drops star anise essential oil
* Fractionated coconut oil or other carrier oil

Add the essential oils to an empty 10-milliliter rollerball bottle. Top it up with fractionated coconut oil, and replace the rollerball top and cap. Gently shake until well combined. Apply to your abdomen and wrists twice daily for at least one month. Inhale deeply each time you use the blend.

DR. COOK'S ESTROGEN-BOOSTING BLEND

Whether you're suffering from PMS, low estrogen levels, or amenorrhea, you'll find this blend a relaxing, gentle healer that boosts mood and has a euphoric effect.

Yield: 1 (10-milliliter) bottle

* 15 drops clary sage essential oil
* 5 drops niaouli essential oil
* 5 drops peppermint essential oil
* 5 drops star anise essential oil
* Fractionated coconut oil or other carrier oil

Add the essential oils to an empty 10-milliliter rollerball bottle and top up the bottle with fractionated coconut oil. Replace the rollerball and top and gently shake until well combined. Apply to your inner wrists, neck, or abdomen two to three times daily.

7 Things to Know Before You Pop the Pill

The Pill is well-known as a form of contraception, but it is also frequently used by the medical profession as a way to "balance" hormones.

However, birth control pills never actually address the root cause of your hormonal or health issues. It is merely a Band-Aid attempt to stop symptoms, but when you eventually go off the Pill, the hormone imbalances will simply come back and often come back worse than before you started, and you may even develop new symptoms. They turn off the connection between the brain and our hormones, which is not something we should ever strive for or accept as normal. They deplete nutrients, throw off gut health, and disrupt brain chemistry.

Regardless of the safety issues, some women will undoubtedly take the Pill or be instructed by their doctors to take the Pill. If you are going to use it, there are some important considerations:

1. Smoking and the Pill don't mix. Women who smoke tobacco and use oral contraceptives have a five-times greater risk of dying from a heart attack than oral contraceptive users who don't smoke. The risk of death linked to circulatory disease is greatly increased in women over the age of 35 who smoke and use oral contraceptives. Avoiding or quitting smoking while using oral contraceptives is recommended.

2. Oral contraceptives can cause folic acid depletion, which can cause a wide variety of health issues from fatigue to abnormal cervical cell growth.

3. The Pill may increase iron levels. Because menstrual blood loss is reduced while using oral contraceptives, iron stores may increase, lessening the need for iron in premenopausal women. Iron levels should be monitored by a physician in women taking oral contraceptives and before taking iron-containing supplements since excess iron has been linked to heart disease.

4. The Pill may deplete magnesium. Women using oral contraceptives were found in studies to have lower levels of magnesium than non-users of this drug. Supplementation of 250–350 milligrams of magnesium per day may be beneficial for women taking oral contraceptives.

5. Oral contraceptives are also associated with vitamin B_6 depletion and clinical depression.

6. The Pill may cause depletion of many other nutrients, including vitamins B_1, B_2, B_3, B_{12}, C, and zinc. The drugs may also interfere with manganese absorption. All of these vitamins and minerals are essential for energy, balanced moods, hormonal health, immune system strength, and many other bodily functions.

7. Don't mix the Pill with the herb St. John's wort since the two may interact, causing changes in menstrual bleeding. Women taking oral contraceptives should consult a physician or qualified herbal practitioner before using St. John's wort.

Are You Suffering from Estrogen Dominance?

Sometimes estrogen levels can become too high relative to the levels of the hormone progesterone. This condition is called estrogen dominance.

There are many reasons why you may be suffering from high estrogen levels. Exposure to xenoestrogens can cause major hormone imbalances, in both men and women. Xenoestrogens mimic the body's own estrogen but are much stronger than human estrogen, which throws off the body's delicate hormonal balance. Candida infections may also play a role, as candida yeast can secrete estrogen-like toxins. Health conditions such as liver disease, low levels of progesterone (which I'll discuss more momentarily), obesity, and ovarian tumors can affect estrogen levels. There are also medications that can increase estrogen levels in your body, including contraceptives, some antibiotics, and phenothiazines, which are used for some emotional disorders.

Estrogen dominance can be linked to a wide variety of symptoms, including the following:

* Anxiety
* Bloating
* Cold hands and feet
* Depression
* Difficulty sleeping
* Fatigue
* Hair loss
* Headaches
* Heavy bleeding
* Irregular periods
* Light spotting
* Low libido
* Memory problems
* Non-cancerous breast lumps
* Severe PMS
* Swollen or tender breasts
* Uterine fibroids

Men can also suffer from excess estrogen. Their symptoms typically include:

* Enlarged breasts or gynecomastia
* Erectile dysfunction
* Infertility

The best ways to address estrogen dominance are to reduce your exposure to plastics and harmful toxic chemicals that have estrogen activity (see page 144 for more information), use antibiotics only when necessary, and avoid using chemical contraceptives. Improving the health of your liver (as discussed on page 21) and losing excess weight through healthy eating and exercise will also help you feel better, as will increasing your levels of progesterone. Don't forget to consult your physician to determine if there are any options other than phenothiazines or other medications you may be taking, and to rule out serious health conditions like ovarian tumors or liver disease.

Restore Your Progesterone Levels

In addition to addressing imbalances in estrogen levels, you may also need to address low levels of the hormone progesterone. As we learned earlier, progesterone is a natural hormone that is primarily manufactured by a woman's ovaries following ovulation in her monthly cycle. Many women suffer from low levels of this hormone for a number of reasons including exposure to a growing number of xenoestrogens in our food, air, and water. Progesterone and estrogen work together to help keep each other in balance. That's why women with low progesterone levels often have high estrogen. Sometimes, simply getting the progesterone levels higher can help lower estrogen levels. When xenoestrogens unnaturally raise estrogen to high levels, this can, in turn, also throw off progesterone levels.

Are You Suffering from Low Progesterone Levels?

There are many signs or symptoms of low levels of progesterone, which include:

* Allergies or asthma
* Autoimmune disease or hives
* Difficulty falling or staying asleep
* Dry skin or sagging skin
* Feeling cold and/or cold hands or feet
* Fibrocystic breast disease
* Hair loss
* Headaches or migraines
* Heart palpitations
* Hot flashes
* Infertility or absent menstruation (not linked to being menopausal)
* Irritability and/or anxiety
* Lack of sweating
* Loss of bone density or osteoporosis
* Low libido
* Menopause
* Premenstrual syndrome with these specific symptoms: breast tenderness, anxiety, sleep disruptions, headaches, menstrual spotting, water retention, bloating, or weight gain
* Prostate enlargement (in men)
* Short menstrual cycle (less than 28 days) or extremely long bleeding times (more than 6 days)
* Varicose or spider veins
* Water retention

Essential Oils to Boost Progesterone Levels

While there are fewer essential oils that can boost progesterone levels than can boost estrogen, there are still some excellent and promising options.

GERANIUM
(Pelargonium graveolens)

This delightfully smelling essential oil can offer more than just a sensual massage experience; it can also help restore healthy hormone levels at the same time, including progesterone levels.

GRAPEFRUIT
(Citrus × paradisi)

Grapefruit essential oil is mood-enhancing and energy boosting, and freshens the smell of any room in which it is used. It is also a good essential oil to help restore healthy progesterone levels. Use internally in capsules or in juice or water for this purpose.

OREGANO
(Origanum vulgare)

Best known for its anti-viral and anti-bacterial activity, oregano essential oil can also help to restore healthy progesterone levels in the body, particularly when added to empty capsules and taken internally.

THYME
(Thymus vulgaris)

Like oregano, thyme is a powerful antimicrobial essential oil that is best known for its ability to fight viral, bacterial, and fungal infections, but it is also a good choice to boost progesterone levels in the body, when used in capsules and taken internally.

TURMERIC
(Curcuma longal)

This brilliant yellow Indian essential oil is a powerful anti-inflammatory that may help restore healthy hormone levels, and seems to balance both progesterone and estrogen levels.

Looking for More Help?

✳ Low progesterone levels can make you feel tired. Feel more energized with the help of the oils on page 68.

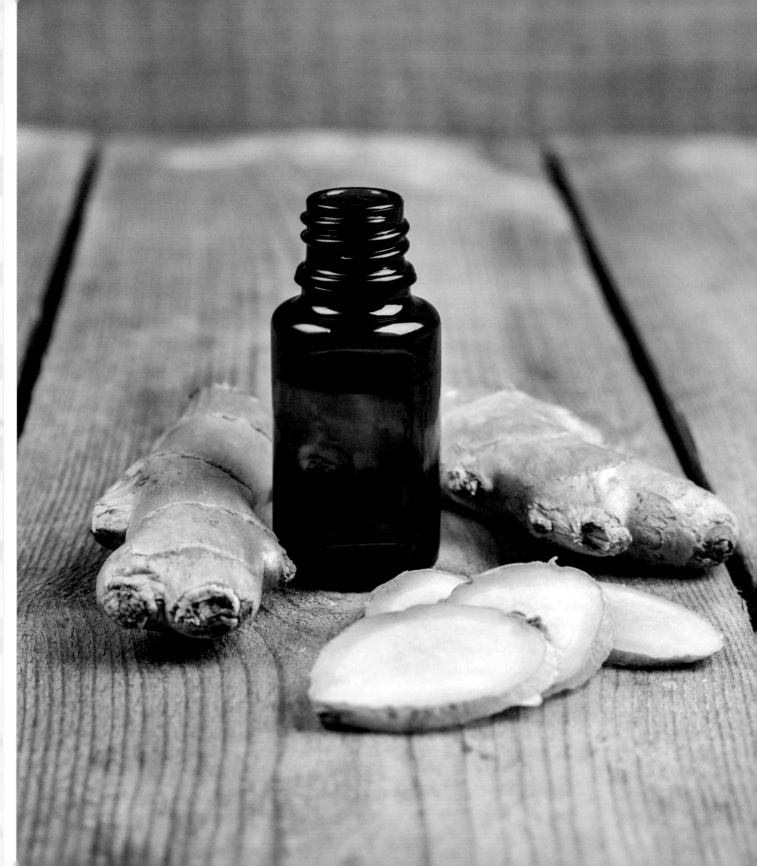

7

The Male Rebuild

The DIY Hormone Solution
for Men's
Vigor and Vitality

W HEN IT COMES TO HORMONES, FEW PEOPLE consider the way they may be affecting men's health. But men also experience hormonal influences that may be impacting their quality of life and vitality.

The primary sexual organs in men comprise the penis and testes. The latter produce sperm as well as the hormone testosterone. In addition to the testes, both men and women's adrenal glands also produce testosterone (check out chapter 3 for more information on the adrenals and boosting their function).

Essential Oils for Thinning Hair

It might be hard to imagine that essential oils can help regrow thinning hair, but fortunately, research shows that they can. And I witnessed it firsthand when a woman in my Medical Aromatherapy essential oil group took before and after photos of her husband's scalp when he used rosemary essential oil. It was surprising how much more hair had grown back. So, if you're suffering from thinning hair, you'll definitely want to give these oils a try. You'll need to be diligent in applying the blend every day and stick with it for at least a few months to get results, but those who do are always glad they stuck with it.

BERGAMOT
(Citrus bergamia)

In a study published in the journal *Food Science & Nutrition*, researchers found that bergamot essential oil was helpful for promoting hair growth. Dilute it in a carrier oil and apply it to affected areas for best results.

CEDARWOOD, LAVENDER, ROSEMARY, AND THYME
(Cedrus atlantica), (Lavandula angustifolia), (Rosmarinus officinalis), (Thymus vulgaris)

Research published in the *International Journal of Pharmaceutical Sciences and Research* found that the combination of these essential oils is beneficial for hair regrowth. To reap the benefits of these oils, add 10 drops of each oil to 10 milliliters of coconut oil and massage it into your scalp on a daily basis for several months.

ROSEMARY
(Rosmarinus officinalis)

Additional research found that rosemary, in particular, is highly effective at increasing hair regrowth and reducing hair loss, especially if it is caused by excessive testosterone. In an article published in the journal *Phytotherapy Research*, scientists found that applying an extract made of rosemary improved hair regrowth in animals affected by excess amounts of testosterone. Scientists observed that the rosemary extract appears to block dihydrotestosterone, an active form of testosterone, from binding to androgen receptor sites. In doing so, rosemary encouraged hair regrowth.

DR. COOK'S SCIENCE-BASED HAIR REGROWTH FORMULA

While there are many chemical hair regrowth formulas on the market, they may not all be safe for long-term use. This blend is made up of research-tested essential oils that can potentially boost hair growth. Daily applications to the scalp are critical to its success.

Yield: 1 (10-milliliter) bottle

* 5 drops bergamot essential oil
* 5 drops cedarwood essential oil
* 5 drops lavender essential oil
* 10 drops rosemary essential oil
* 5 drops thyme essential oil
* Fractionated coconut oil or other carrier oil

In a 10-milliliter rollerball bottle, combine the essential oils. Top up the bottle with fractionated coconut oil or another carrier oil until full. Gently shake the bottle until the oils are combined. Apply to your scalp every evening before bed.

HAIR LOSS SOLUTION

Add the following oils to your natural hair conditioner to help it boost hair growth and prevent hair loss.

Yield: 1 bottle

* 10 drops bergamot essential oil
* 10 drops cedarwood essential oil
* 30 drops rosemary essential oil

Add the essential oils to your favorite 250-milliliter bottle of natural hair conditioner. Shake until combined. Apply a dollop of conditioner, massaging it into your scalp for at least one minute daily before rinsing.

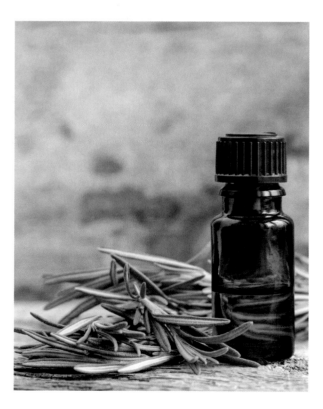

Essential Oils to Boost Your Libido

Whether you're suffering from a low libido due to insufficient testosterone or poor adrenal health, essential oils can help. This is true for both men and women. In addition to boosting sensual pleasure due to their heavenly aromas, essential oils can help boost your libido and act as natural aphrodisiacs to maximize sexual pleasure.

GINGER
(Zingiber officinale)

Not only does ginger taste great in our baking and cooking, it is also a natural libido booster. Research shows that regular ingestion or supplementation with gingerroot can boost testosterone levels, which are imperative for a healthy sex drive in men as well as women. Of course, the essential oil extract of gingerroot can have the same effect.

ROSE
(Rosa damascena)

Toxins in our environment can take their toll on our hormonal health. Research shows that regular inhalation of rose essential oil can help protect male sexual health from damage, particularly due to formaldehyde toxicity. Because rose can protect testosterone levels, which are essential to a healthy sex drive, it may boost libido.

YLANG-YLANG
(Cananga odorata)

Used for centuries as a natural aphrodisiac, ylang-ylang is also believed to reduce sexual anxiety, making it an ideal choice if you're suffering with a low libido or any anxiety linked to consensual sex.

Low testosterone levels are often behind a low sex drive. Whether you are a woman or man, you may find it beneficial to give your testosterone levels a boost.

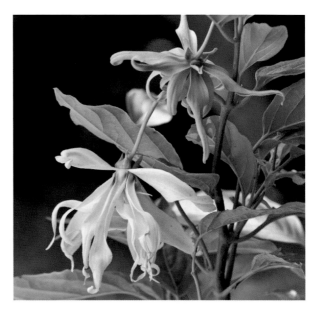

Essential Oils for an Active Lifestyle

While the bulk of my practice over the years has been working with women, helping them to address their health needs, the majority of men who sought my help often did so to improve their athletic performance. This is an area that is just as important for women, but it is also a great way for many men to launch their interest in using natural remedies to improve their health and life.

There are so many great health reasons to stay active, but let's face it: sometimes there are a few bumps, bruises, and bugs along the way. Fortunately, essential oils can help. Here are some of the best essential oils to keep on hand for an active lifestyle:

COPAIBA
(Copaifera reticulata, C. officinalis, C. coriacea, and C. langsdorffii)

Copaiba's beta-caryophyllene shows great promise in the treatment of joint pain. A study published in the *Journal of Cellular Biochemistry* found that copaiba demonstrated potent anti-inflammatory activity throughout the body and also reduced the number of free radicals that tend to be involved in the degradation of joints, making it a great choice for an active lifestyle and the joint pain that sometimes accompanies it.

GINGER
(Zingiber officinale)

Ginger is not just delicious in food, it is also a powerful essential oil that, when diluted and applied topically to the skin, stimulates circulation in the joints, alleviates stiffness, warms the muscles and joints, and helps reduce pain. You need to dilute it in a carrier oil before using, and avoid it if you have highly sensitive skin.

LAVENDER
(Lavandula angustifolia)

Lavender is great for speeding the healing of sunburns and easing the discomfort they cause. Simply put a drop of lavender oil diluted in five drops of coconut oil or other carrier oil on burns to speed healing and ease the burn pain.

LEMON EUCALYPTUS
(Eucalyptus citriodora)

If your active lifestyle keeps you spending time outdoors, you'll want an essential oil that will keep the mosquitoes and other pesky bugs at bay. But, you'll want to skip the toxic bug repellents that smell disgusting and contain harmful DEET. Choose lemon eucalyptus essential oil instead. A study published in the *Journal of the American Mosquito Control Association* found that lemon eucalyptus was highly effective against mosquitoes. Another study in the *Journal of Insect Science* study found that a product made up of lemon eucalyptus outperformed almost all DEET-based insect repellents with its 91 percent repellency rate.

MARJORAM
(Origanum majorana)

Marjoram oil is particularly good for easing tight muscles, which is a common issue when enlisting lesser-used muscles during and after workouts. Apply marjoram to inflamed joints to help ease inflammation. Additionally, you'll love marjoram if your workout takes you outdoors. A study published in *Natural Products Research* found that marjoram was as effective as DEET-based insecticides at repelling mosquitoes. It is also highly effective at repelling ticks, making it an excellent choice when your active life takes you to wooded areas. Avoid use during pregnancy or if you suffer from epilepsy.

YLANG-YLANG
(Cananga odorata)

A study published in the journal *Parasitology Research* found that ylang-ylang essential oil repelled 97.1 to 99.4 percent of various species of mosquitoes. Compare that to the findings of the *Journal of Insect Science* study mentioned earlier, which showed the DEET-based OFF Deep Woods Insect Repellent repelled 94 percent of mosquitoes; Repel 100, made up of 98.11 percent DEET, only had a 90 percent repellency rate; and Avon Skin-So-Soft Bug Guard only repelled 52 percent of mosquitoes.

DIY MOSQUITO REPELLENT

If you're spending much time outdoors, you know how pesky mosquitoes can be. Fortunately, the following mosquito repellent is highly effective at repelling the little pests.

Yield: 1 (30-milliliter) bottle

* 30 drops lemon eucalyptus essential oil
* 15 drops marjoram essential oil
* 15 drops ylang-ylang essential oil
* Fractionated coconut oil or other carrier oil

In an empty 30-milliliter bottle, add the essential oils. Top up with fractionated coconut oil. Replace the top and gently shake to combine ingredients. Apply every few hours or as needed to skin to keep mosquitoes at bay.

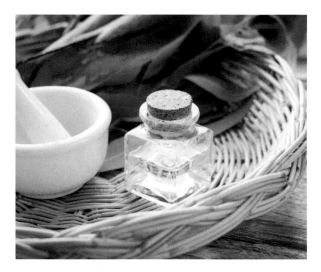

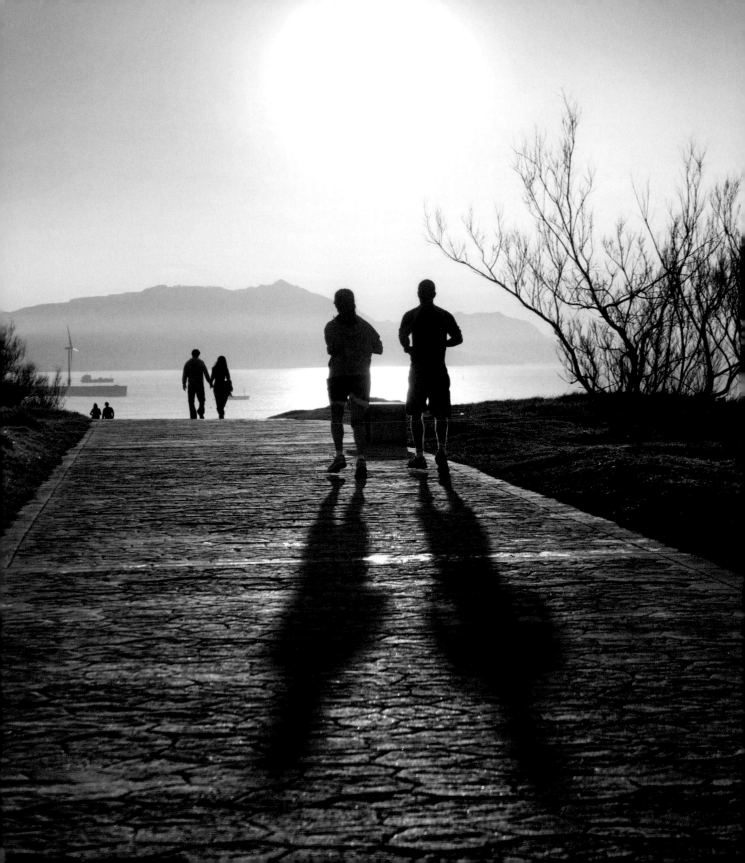

Essential Oil Usage Chart

This chart outlines the uses for the top essential oils that address the hormone-related conditions described in the book. Remember, if you're planning to use any oils internally, choose only the highest-quality products that indicate their suitability for internal use on the label. If you are pregnant or breastfeeding, please note research about the safety of essential oils for use during these times changes. Any essential oils should be used with caution and the approval of a physician during pregnancy or breastfeeding

ESSENTIAL OIL	DIFFUSE	TOPICAL	INTERNAL	PRECAUTIONS
Basil	✔	✔	✔	Dilute for topical use. If pregnant or breastfeeding, use with the guidance of a physician.
Bergamot	✔	✔	✔	Dilute for topical use. Avoid direct sunlight or UV rays for at least twelve hours after topical application. If pregnant or breastfeeding, use with the guidance of a physician.
Black spruce	✔	✔		Use externally only.
Blue tansy	✔	✔		Dilute for topical use. Avoid use during pregnancy or breastfeeding. May stain surfaces and fabrics.
Cedarwood	✔	✔		Dilute for topical use. If pregnant or breastfeeding, use with the guidance of a physician.
Chamomile (Roman chamomile and German chamomile)	✔	✔		Avoid using chamomile if you have an allergy to ragweed or if you are using blood-thinning drugs, especially warfarin.
Cinnamon	✔	✔	✔	Dilute for topical and internal use. Use in an empty capsule for internal use.
Clary sage	✔	✔		Use with caution during the first two trimesters of pregnancy.
Clove	✔	✔	✔	Dilute for topical and internal use. If pregnant or breastfeeding or if you are suffering from a liver condition, use with the guidance of a physician.
Copaiba	✔	✔	✔	Dilute for topical use if you have sensitive skin.
Coriander	✔	✔	✔	None.
Cypress	✔	✔		Use externally only.

ESSENTIAL OIL	DIFFUSE	TOPICAL	INTERNAL	PRECAUTIONS
Eucalyptus	✔	✔		Dilute for topical use if you have sensitive skin.
Fennel	✔	✔	✔	Dilute for topical use. If pregnant or breastfeeding, use with the guidance of a physician. Do not use if you have epilepsy or seizures.
Frankincense	✔	✔	✔	Dilute for topical use if you have sensitive skin.
Geranium	✔	✔		Dilute for topical use if you have sensitive skin.
Ginger	✔	✔	✔	Dilute for topical use. Use in empty capsules for internal use.
Grapefruit	✔	✔	✔	Dilute for topical use if you have sensitive skin. Avoid direct sun exposure and UV rays for at least 12 hours after topical application. While some prescription drugs warn against grapefruit consumption to avoid potential drug interactions, the warning does not seem to apply to grapefruit essential oil, which has a different chemical composition than the fruit.
Helichrysum	✔	✔	✔	Do not use during pregnancy.
Jasmine	✔	✔		Most jasmine essential oils on the market are extracted with chemical solvents, which may spoil any medicinal value they offer; these are best avoided.
Juniper	✔	✔	✔	Do not use during pregnancy.
Lavender	✔	✔	✔	Dilute for topical use if you have sensitive skin.
Lemon	✔	✔	✔	Dilute for topical use if you have sensitive skin. Avoid sun exposure and UV rays within 12 hours of topical application.
Lemon eucalyptus	✔	✔		Dilute for topical use if you have sensitive skin.
Lemongrass	✔	✔	✔	Dilute for topical use.
Marjoram	✔	✔	✔	Use with caution during the first trimester of pregnancy.
Melissa	✔	✔	✔	Most of the oil sold as melissa essential oil is not actually extracted from *Melissa officinalis*; it is typically a blend of lemongrass and citronella, as well as other chemicals, and is best avoided.

ESSENTIAL OIL	DIFFUSE	TOPICAL	INTERNAL	PRECAUTIONS
Myrrh	✔	✔	✔	Avoid use during pregnancy or breastfeeding.
Niaouli	✔	✔		Use with caution if pregnant and breastfeeding.
Oregano	✔	✔	✔	Dilute for topical and internal use. Use in an empty capsule for internal use. Use with caution during pregnancy.
Orange (sweet orange and wild orange)	✔	✔	✔	Dilute for topical use if you have sensitive skin. Avoid sun exposure and UV rays within 12 hours of topical application.
Peppermint	✔	✔	✔	Safe to apply undiluted; however, use only 1 or 2 drops at a time as it has potent cooling effects. Be careful not to diffuse too much peppermint essential oil as the fumes may cause your eyes to water. Avoid getting the oil in your eyes, and be sure to wash your hands immediately after use to prevent rubbing the peppermint oil into your eyes.
Pine	✔	✔		Dilute for topical use. May irritate sensitive skin.
Rose	✔	✔		Most of the rose essential oil on the market has been cut with cheaper oils, solvents, carrier oils, and lesser species of the plant. If the oil you're buying is inexpensive, it is unlikely to be pure enough for therapeutic use.
Rose geranium	✔	✔		Dilute for topical use if you have sensitive skin.
Rosemary	✔	✔	✔	Do not use during pregnancy or if you have epilepsy.
Sandalwood	✔	✔	✔	None.
Spearmint	✔	✔	✔	None.
Star anise	✔	✔		Dilute for topical use.
Tarragon	✔	✔	✔	Dilute for topical use.
Tea tree	✔	✔	✔	Dilute for topical use if you have sensitive skin.
Thyme	✔	✔	✔	Dilute for topical and internal use. Use in an empty capsule for internal use. Use with caution during pregnancy or if you have epilepsy or high blood pressure.

ESSENTIAL OIL	DIFFUSE	TOPICAL	INTERNAL	PRECAUTIONS
Turmeric	✔	✔	✔	Dilute for topical use.
Vetiver	✔	✔		Use externally only.
Wintergreen	✔	✔		Use externally only. Dilute for topical use. Sadly, most "wintergreen" oil on the market is now synthetic, has no medicinal value, and may actually be harmful. Check the label for dosage information. If it does not contain this information, then it is not suitable for internal use.
Ylang-ylang	✔	✔		Use externally only.

ACKNOWLEDGMENTS

To Curtis, for always believing in me, loving me, for everything you do to treat me like a queen, and for picking up the slack around our home and acreage as I wrote this book.

To my sister, Bobbi-Jo Meyer, and mom, Deborah Schoffro, for all your support and encouragement with my work in essential oils.

To my dear old Dad, Michael Schoffro, for everything you do and for being such a great dad.

To Jane Mullin and Angela Grow, for all your support for my work with essential oils.

To the wonderful and unmatched team of baristas at the Kemptville Starbucks, for cheering me on, helping to keep my mind sharp with your witticisms, providing me with fuel, and for your friendship and support as I became your self-appointed writer-in-residence.

To my team of amazing women and men who have chosen to share their journey with essential oils with me.

To the team at Sterling, for your belief in this project and your excellent work to turn it into the lovely book it has become.

To Regina Brooks at Serendipity Literary Agency, for your belief in this project and for your efforts to find it a good home.

NOTES

 What's Going on with Me?:
Dr. Cook's 10-Day Plan for Hormone Perfection

14 **"There are many other signs"**: Xandria Williams, *The Herbal Detox Plan: The Revolutionary Way to Cleanse and Revive Your Body* (Carlsbad, CA: Hay House, 2004), 83; Gloria Gilbere, "A Doctor's Solution to 'Plumbing Problems' in Your Gut That Is!," *Total Health* 26, no. 1 (February 2004), 37.

16 **"In one study, researchers found"**: S. Yagi et al., "Chemical composition, anti-proliferative, antioxidant, and antibacterial activities of essential oils from aromatic plants growing in Sudan," *Asian Pacific Journal of Tropical Medicine* 8 (August 2016): 763–70, https://www.ncbi.nlm.nih.gov/pubmed/27569885.

16 **"Other research in *Letters in Applied Microbiology* journal"**: D. Schillaci et al., "In vitro anti-biofilm activity of Boswellia spp. Oleogum resin essential oils," *Letters in Applied Microbiology* 47, no. 5 (November 2008), 43–48. https://www.ncbi.nlm.nih.gov/pubmed/19146534.

16 **"While the study was conducted"**: S. Ribel-Madsen et al., "A synoviocyte model for osteoarthritis and rheumatoid arthritis: response to ibuprofen, betamethasone, and ginger extract—a cross-sectional in vitro study," *Arthritis* (2012). https://www.ncbi.nlm.nih.gov/pubmed/23365744.

16 **"A study published in the *Journal of Natural Products*"**: J. Zhao et al., "Octulosonic acid derivatives from Roman chamomile (*Chamaemelum nobile*) with activities against inflammation and metabolic disorder," *Journal of Natural Products* 77, no. 3 (March 28, 2014): 509–15. https://www.ncbi.nlm.nih.gov/pubmed/24471493.

17 **"Many studies demonstrate"**: B. B. Aggarwal et al., "Curcumin-free turmeric exhibits anti-inflammatory and anti-cancer activities: Identification of novel components in turmeric," *Molecular Nutrition & Food Research* 57, no. 9 (September 2013): 1529–42. https://www.ncbi.nlm.nih.gov/pubmed/23847105.

18 **"Research in the journal *Molecules*"**: M. Sienkiewicz et al., "The potential use of basil and rosemary essential oils as effective antibacterial agents," *Molecules* 18, no. 8 (August 5, 2013): 9334–51. https://www.ncbi.nlm.nih.gov/pubmed/23921795.

18 **"According to a preliminary study"**: A. Gemechu et al., "In vitro anti-mycobacterial activity of selected medicinal plants against *Mycobacterium tuberculosis* and *Mycobacterium bovis* strains," *BMC Complementary and Alternative Medicine* 13 (October 29, 2013): 291. https://www.ncbi.nlm.nih.gov/pubmed/24168665.

18 **"Researchers assessed the antimicrobial activity"**: "What is Chamomile?" WebMD. https://www.webmd.com/diet/supplement-guide-chamomile#1.

18 **"This study could help explain"**: H. Rahman and A. Chandra, "Microbiologic evaluation of matricaria and chlorhexidine against *E. faecalis* and *C. albicans*," *Indian Journal of Dentistry* 6, no. 2 (April–June 2015): 60–64. https://www.ncbi.nlm.nih.gov/pubmed/26097333.

18 **"In a study published in *BMC Complementary and Alternative Medicine*"**: R. Naveed et al., "Antimicrobial activity of the bioactive components of essential oils from Pakistani spices against Salmonella and other multi-drug resistant bacteria.," *BMC Complementary and Alternative Medicine* 13 (October 14, 2013): 265. https://www.ncbi.nlm.nih.gov/pubmed/24119438.

19 **"But, rose is a powerful"**: S. Ulusoy et al., "Tocopherol, carotene, phenolic contents and antibacterial properties of rose essential oil, hydrosol, and absolute," *Current Microbiology* 59, no. 5 (November 2009): 554–58.

19 **"Research in the *Journal of Antimicrobial Chemotherapy*"**: G. K. F. Elsom and D. Hide, "Susceptibility of methicillin-resistant *Staphylococcus aureus* to tea tree oil and mupiricin," *Journal of Antimicrobial Chemotherapy* 43, no. 3 (March 1, 1999): 427–28. https://academic.oup.com/jac/article/43/3/427/755098.

19 **"Other research published in the *International Journal of Antimicrobial Agents*"**: Jakub Kwiecinski et al., "Effects of Tea Tree (Melaleuca alternifolia) oil on *Staphylococcus aureus* in biofilms and stationary growth phase," *International Journal of Antimicrobial Agents* 33, no. 4 (April 2009): 343–7. https://www.sciencedirect.com/science/article/abs/pii/S0924857908004445.

19 **"In a review of thyme"**: Hercules Sakkas and Chrissanthy Papadopoulou, "Antimicrobial activity of basil, oregano, and thyme essential oils," *Journal of Microbiology and Biotechnology* 27, no. 3 (2017), 429–38. http://www.jmb.or.kr/submission/Journal/027/JMB027-03-02_FDOC_1.pdf.

21 **"The average person consumes fourteen pounds"**: Frances Albrecht, "The Basics of Detoxing Your Liver," Healthwell, April 1997.

23 **"Research in the *British Journal of Nutrition*"**: M. A. Calleja et al., "The antioxidant effect of β-caryophyllene protects rat liver from carbon tetrachloride-induced fibrosis by inhibiting hepatic stellate cell activation," *British Journal of Nutrition* 109, no. 3 (February 14, 2013): 394–401. https://www.ncbi.nlm.nih.gov/pubmed/22717234.

23 **"Research in the journal *Frontiers in Pharmacology*"**: K. Loeser et al., "Protective effect of Casperone, an orally bioavailable frankincense extract, on lipopolysaccharide-induced systemic inflammation in mice," *Frontiers in Pharmacology* 9 (April 20, 2018): 387. https://www.ncbi.nlm.nih.gov/pubmed/29731716.

24 **"Research in the journal *BMC Complementary and Alternative Medicine*"**: A. Raskovic et al., "Antioxidant activity of rosemary (Rosmarinus officinalis L.) essential oil and its hepatoprotective potential," *BMC Complementary and Alternative Medicine* 14 (July 7, 2014): 225. https://www.ncbi.nlm.nih.gov/pubmed/25002023.

24 **"Research in the journal *Biofactors*"**: P. G. Bradford, "Curcumin and obesity," *Biofactors* 39, no. 1 (January–February 2013): 78–87. https://www.ncbi.nlm.nih.gov/pubmed/23339049.

28 **"The study also found that the higher the added sugar intake"**: Quanhe Yang et al, "Added sugar intake and cardiovascular diseases mortality among US adults," *JAMA Network*, April 2014. https://jamanetwork.com/journals/jamainternalmedicine/fullarticle/1819573.

28 **"Do You Have Excess Insulin?"**: Natasha Turner, *The Hormone Diet: A 3-Step Program to Help You Lose Weight, Gain Strength, and Live Younger Longer*. New York: Rodale, 2010, 40–41.

30 **"It is often a precursor to diabetes"**: S. Gupta Jain et al., "Effect of oral cinnamon intervention on metabolic profile and body composition of Asian Indians with metabolic syndrome: a randomized, double-blind control trial," *Lipids in Health and Disease* 16, no. 1 (June 12, 2017): 113. https://www.ncbi.nlm.nih.gov/pubmed/28606084.

30 **"While testing of this essential oil"**: Rafie Hamdipour et al., "Chemistry, pharmacology, and medicinal property of sage (*Salvia*) to prevent and cure illnesses such as obesity, diabetes, depression, dementia, lupus, autism, heart disease, and cancer," *Global Journal of Medical Research: Pharma, Drug Discovery, Toxicology, and Medicine* 13, no. 7 (2013). https://globaljournals.org/GJMR_Volume13/1-Chemistry-Pharmacology.pdf.

30 **"Researchers have found that ginger"**: Nafiseh Shokri Mashhadi et al., "Anti-oxidative and anti-inflammatory effects of ginger in health and physical activity: review of current evidence," *International Journal of Preventive Medicine* 4, Supplement 1 (April 2013): S36–S42. https://www.ncbi.nlm.nih.gov/pmc/articles/PMC3665023/.

30 **"Research shows that rats"**: Jon Johnson, "9 Essential Oils for Diabetes," Medical News Today, April 20, 2017. https://www.medicalnewstoday.com/articles/317017.php.

30 **"Exposure to the scent"**: Kaitlyn Berkheiser, "6 Benefits and Uses of Grapefruit Essential Oil," Healthline. https://www.healthline.com/nutrition/grapefruit-essential-oil#section1.

31 **"While there is little research testing"**: Henda Keskes et al., "In vitro anti-diabetic, anti-obesity, and antioxidant properties of *Juniperus phoenicia* L. leaves from Tunisia," *Asian Pacific Journal of Tropical Biomedicine* 4, Supplement 2 (July 2014): S649–655. https://www.sciencedirect.com/science/article/pii/S2221169115300654.

31 **"In a study of exercise performance"**: A. Mearmarbashi and A. Rajabi, "The effects of peppermint on exercise performance," *Journal of the International Society of Sports Nutrition* 10, no. 1 (March 21, 2003): 15. https://www.ncbi.nlm.nih.gov/pubmed/23517650/.

32 **"BHA has been linked to cancer"**: "The Dirty Dozen: BHA and BHT," David Suzuki Foundation. https://davidsuzuki.org/queen-of-green/dirty-dozen-bha-bht/.

32 **"They can cause liver"**: "The Dirty Dozen: DEA-related ingredients," David Suzuki Foundation. https://davidsuzuki.org/queen-of-green/the-dirty-dozen-dea-related-ingredients/.

32 **"Used as a solvent for dyes"**: "The Dirty Dozen: Dibutyl phthalate," David Suzuki Foundation. https://davidsuzuki.org/queen-of-green/dirty-dozen-dibutyl-phthalate/.

32 **"In a study published in the journal *Environmental Research*"**: J. Axelsson et al., "Prenatal phthalate exposure and reproductive function in young men," *Environmental Research* 138 (April 2015): 264–70. https://www.ncbi.nlm.nih.gov/pubmed/25743932.

32 **"In another animal study"**: N. Sen et al., "Short-term exposure to di-n-butyl phthalate disrupts ovarian function in young CD-1 mice," *Reproductive Toxicology* 53 (June 2015): 15–22. https://www.ncbi.nlm.nih.gov/pubmed/25765776.

33 **"You'll find them in body care products"**: "The Dirty Dozen: Parfum (aka ""Fragrance"")," David Suzuki Foundation. https://davidsuzuki.org/queen-of-green/dirty-dozen-parfum-fragrance/.

33 **"Parabens in cosmetics"**: "The Dirty Dozen: Parabens," David Suzuki Foundation. https://davidsuzuki.org/queen-of-green/dirty-dozen-parabens/.

33 **"They are toxic to the reproductive system"**: "The Dirty Dozen: Siloxanes," David Suzuki Foundation. https://davidsuzuki.org/queen-of-green/dirty-dozen-siloxanes/.

33 **"Dr. Gaurab Chakrabarti, MD, PhD, at the Philadelphia-based biotechnology company"**: Gaurab Chakrabarti, "Which Cleaning Products are Polluting Your Home the Most?" Ode to Clean, January 2, 2018. https://odetoclean.com/blogs/fresh-air/which-cleaning-products-are-polluting-your-home-the-most.

33 **"VOCs are gasses that enter the air"**: "Cheat Sheet: Volatile organic compounds," Environmental Working Group, May 14, 2008. https://www.ewg.org/enviroblog/2008/05/cheatsheet-volatile-organic-compounds#.WpBz-BrQdPY.

33 **"VOCs have been found"**: "Cheat Sheet: Volatile organic compounds," Environmental Working Group, May 14, 2008. https://www.ewg.org/enviroblog/2008/05/cheatsheet-volatile-organic-compounds#.WpBz-BrQdPY.

34 **"In research published in the journal *Environmental Health*"**: G. D. Bittner et al., "Estrogenic chemicals often leach from BPA-free plastic products that are replacements for BPA-containing polycarbonate products," *Environmental Health* 13, no. 1 (May 28, 2014): 41. https://www.ncbi.nlm.nih.gov/pubmed/24886603.

34 **"Teflon, also known as perfluorooctanoic acid"**: Bill Walker and David Andrews, "Teflon Chemical Unsafe at Smallest Doses: EPA's 'Safe' Level is Hundreds or Thousands of Times Too Weak," Environmental Working Group, August 2015. http://static.ewg.org/reports/2015/pfoa_drinking_water/Teflon_Chemical_Unsafe_At_Small_Doses_.pdf?_ga=1.123867018.1229808912.1430957370.

3   Adrenal Rejuvenation: Restore Your Energy and Vitality

57 **"Insulin resistance usually causes"**: William C. Shiel Jr., MD, FACP, FACR, "Medical Definition of Insulin Resistance," MedicineNet. https://www.medicinenet.com/script/main/art.asp?articlekey=18822.

57 **"Do You Have Excess Cortisol?"**: Natasha Turner, ND, *The Hormone Diet: A 3-Step Program to Help You Lose Weight, Gain Strength, and Live Younger Longer*. New York: Rodale, 2010, 43.

60 **"The essential oil extracted from cedarwood"**: Eric Zielinski, DC, *The Healing Power of Essential Oils: Soothe Inflammation, Boost Mood, Prevent Autoimmunity, and Feel Great in Every Way*. New York: Harmony Books, 2018, 250.

60 **"The essential oil most known for its hormone-balancing effects"**: G. H. Seol et al., "Antidepressant-like effect of *Salvia sclarea* is explained by modulation of dopamine activities in rats," *Journal of Ethnopharmacology* 130, no. 1 (July 6, 2010): 187–90. https://www.ncbi.nlm.nih.gov/pubmed/20441789.

60 **"In another study of menopausal women"**: K. B. Lee et al., "Changes in 5-hydroxytryptamine and cortisol plasma levels in menopausal women after inhalation of clary sage oil," *Phytotherapy Research* 28, no. 11 (November 2014): 1599–605. https://www.ncbi.nlm.nih.gov/pubmed/24802524.

60 **"Frankincense also contains compounds"**: A. Moussaieff et al., "Incensole acetate reduces depressive-like behavior and modulates hippocampal BDNF and CRF expression of submissive animals," *Journal of Psychopharmacology* 26, no. 12 (December 2012): 1584–93. https://www.ncbi.nlm.nih.gov/pubmed/23015543.

60 **"According to a study in the journal *Behavioural Brain Research*"**: M. Komiya et al., "Lemon oil vapor causes an anti-stress effect via modulating the 5-HT and DA activities in mice," *Behavioural Brain Research* 172, no. 2 (September 25, 2006): 240–49. https://www.ncbi.nlm.nih.gov/pubmed/16780969.

60 **"Research in the *Journal of Agricultural and Food Chemistry*"**: L. L. Zhang, Z. Y. Yang, G. Fan, J. N. Ren, K. J. Yin, and S. Y. Pan, "Antidepressant-like effect of *Citrus sinensis* (L.) Osbeck essential oil and its main component limonene on mice," *Journal of Agricultural and Food Chemistry* 67, no. 50 (April 2 2019): 13817–28. https://www.ncbi.nlm.nih.gov/pubmed/30905156.

62 **"Here are some of the most common signs"**: Kalidasa Brown, "30 Symptoms of Adrenal Fatigue," Natural Healing and Back Pain Relief, July 24, 2016. https://selfadjustingtechnique.com/30-symptoms-of-adrenal-fatigue/.

63 **"In a study published in *Complementary Therapies in Clinical Practice*"**: R. Shirzadegan et al., "Effects of geranium aroma on anxiety among patients with acute myocardial infarction: a triple-blind randomized clinical trial." *Complementary Therapies in Clinical Practice* 29 (November 2017): 201–06. https://www.ncbi.nlm.nih.gov/pubmed/29122262.

64 **"The adrenal cortex makes up"**: William C. Shiel Jr., MD, FACP, FACR, "Medical Definition of Adrenal Cortex," MedicineNet. https://www.medicinenet.com/script/main/art.asp?articlekey=9704.

64 **"Rosemary also contains compounds"**: The George Mateljan Foundation, "Rosemary," WH Foods. http://www.whfoods.com/genpage.php?tname=foodspice&dbid=75.

64 **"Preliminary research in the *Journal of Ethnopharmacology*"**: Nan Zhang et al., "*Cananga odorata* essential oil reverses the anxiety induced by 1-(3-chlorophenyl) piperazine through regulating the MAPK pathway and serotonin system in mice," *Journal of Ethnopharmacology* 219 (June 12, 2018): 23–30. https://www.sciencedirect.com/science/article/pii/S0378874117303483?via%3Dihub.

68 **"Research in the journal *Psychoneuroendocrinology*"**: J. K. Kiecolt-Glasser et al., "Olfactory influences on mood and autonomic, endocrine, and immune function," *Psychoneuroendocrinology* 33, no. 3 (April 2008): 328–29. https://www.ncbi.nlm.nih.gov/pubmed/18178322.

68 **"In a study published in the *Journal of Oleo Science*"**: S. Okano et al., "The effects of frankincense essential oil on stress in rats," *Journal of Oleo Science* 68, no. 10 (2019): 1003–1009. https://www.ncbi.nlm.nih.gov/pubmed/31582666.

68 **"In a study published in the *Journal of the International Society of Sports Nutrition*"**: A. Mearmarbashi and A. Rajabi, "The effects of peppermint on exercise performance," *Journal of the International Society of Sports Nutrition* 10, no. 1 (March 21, 2003): 15. https://www.ncbi.nlm.nih.gov/pubmed/23517650/.

68 **"Another study in the *Journal of the International Society of Sports Nutrition*"**: N. A. Jaradat et al., "The effect of inhalation of *Citrus sinensis* flowers and *Mentha spicata* leave essential oils on lung function and exercise performance: a quasi-experimental uncontrolled before-and-after study," *Journal of the International Society of Sports Nutrition* 13, no. 36 (September 22, 2016): 36. https://www.ncbi.nlm.nih.gov/pubmed/27688737/.

68 **"The study that examined spearmint"**: N. A. Jaradat et al., "The effect of inhalation of *Citrus sinensis* flowers and *Mentha spicata* leave essential oils on lung function and exercise performance: a quasi-experimental uncontrolled before-and-after study," *Journal of the International Society of Sports Nutrition* 13, no. 36 (September 22, 2016): 36. https://www.ncbi.nlm.nih.gov/pubmed/27688737/.

69 **"With a long history of use"**: "Fennel," Our Herb Garden. http://www.ourherbgarden.com/herb-history/fennel.html.

70 **"Research found that ginger's"**: G. Chamani et al., "Evaluation of effects of Zingiber officinale on salivation in rats," *Acta Medica Iranica* 49, no. 6 (2011): 336–40. https://www.ncbi.nlm.nih.gov/pubmed/21874635.

70 **"According to research in the medical journal *Food Science and Biotechnology*"**: Y. Li et al., "In vitro anti-viral, anti-inflammatory, and antioxidant activities of the ethanol extract of Mentha piperita L.," *Food Science and Biotechnology*, 26, no. 6 (November 30, 2017): 1675–83. https://www.ncbi.nlm.nih.gov/pubmed/30263705.

**4 Reset Your Thyroid:
Balance Your Metabolism Even When Nothing Else Works**

81 **"According to the American Association of Clinical Endocrinologists"**: J. Blackwell, "Diagnosis and treatment of hyperthyroidism and hypothyroidism," *Journal of the American Academy of Nurse Practitioners* 16, no. 10 (October 2004): 422–25. https://www.ncbi.nlm.nih.gov/pubmed/15543918.

86 **"It has been found in the journal *Scientific Reports*"**: Su Shulan et al., "Frankincense and myrrh suppress inflammation via regulation of the metabolic profiling and the MAPK signaling pathway," *Scientific Reports* 5 (2014): 13668. https://www.ncbi.nlm.nih.gov/pmc/articles/PMC4556964/.

86 **"Research found that the oil"**: M. N. Boukhatem et al., "Lemongrass (*Cymbopogon citratus*) essential oil as a potent anti-inflammatory and antifungal drugs," *The Libyan Journal of Medicine* 9 (September 19, 2014): 25431. https://www.ncbi.nlm.nih.gov/pubmed/25242268.

86 **"Rose geranium produces"**: Mohammed Nadjib Boukhatem et al., "Rose geranium essential oil as a source of new and safe anti-inflammatory drugs," *Libyan Journal of Medicine* 8 (2013): 22520. https://www.ncbi.nlm.nih.gov/pmc/articles/PMC3793238/.

87 **"In a study published in the medical journal *Endocrine*"**: D. Thomas et al., "Herpes virus antibodies seroprevalence in children with autoimmune thyroid disease," *Endocrine* 33, no. 2 (April 2008): 171–75. https://www.ncbi.nlm.nih.gov/pubmed/18473192.

89 **"Other research at the Department of Nursing"**: H. J. Kim, "Effect of aromatherapy massage on abdominal fat and body image in post-menopausal women," *Taehan Kanho Hakhoe Chi* 37, no. 4 (June 2007): 603–12. https://www.ncbi.nlm.nih.gov/pubmed/17615482.

89 **"In this study, researchers found"**: A. Niijima and K. Nagai, "Effect of olfactory stimulation with flavor of grapefruit oil and lemon oil on the activity of sympathetic branch in the white adipose tissue of the epididymis," *Experimental Biology and Medicine* 228, no. 10 (November 2003): 1190–92.

91 **"Some of the symptoms"**: "What is Hyperthyroidism? What are the Symptoms?" WebMD. https://www.webmd.com/a-to-z-guides/overactive-thyroid-hyperthyroidism.

92 **"While little research has been done":** Kathryn Watson, "Treating Common Thyroid Problems with Essential Oils," Healthline.com. https://www.healthline.com/health/essential-oils-for-thyroid.

92 **"Researchers who have studied lemongrass":** M. N. Boukhatem et al., "Lemongrass (*Cymbopogon citratus*) essential oil as a potent anti-inflammatory and antifungal drugs," *Libyan Journal of Medicine* 9 (September 19, 2014.): 25431. https://www.ncbi.nlm.nih.gov/pubmed/25242268.

92 **"Some research and a lengthy history":** I. Suntar et al., "Appraisal on the wound-healing and anti-inflammatory activities of the essential oils obtained from the cones and needles of the Pinus species by in vivo and in vitro experimental models," *Journal of Ethnopharmacology* 139, no. 2 (January 31, 2012): 533–40. https://www.ncbi.nlm.nih.gov/pubmed/22155393.

92 **"Research published in the medical journal *Worldviews on Evidence-Based Nursing*":** R. Trambert et al., "A randomized-controlled trial provides evidence to support aromatherapy to minimize anxiety in women undergoing breast biopsy," *Worldviews on Evidence-Based Nursing* 14, no. 5 (October 2017): 394–402. https://www.ncbi.nlm.nih.gov/pubmed/28395396.

92 **"Wintergreen essential oil has":** "Methyl salicylate," PubChem. https://pubchem.ncbi.nlm.nih.gov/compound/Methyl-salicylate.

92 **"Research published in the journal *Clinical Therapeutics*":** Y. Higashi et al., "Efficacy and safety profile of a topical methyl salicylate and menthol patch in adult patients with mild to moderate muscle strain: a randomized, double-blind, parallel-group, placebo-controlled, multicenter study," *Clinical Therapeutics* 32, no. 1 (January 2010): 34–43. https://www.ncbi.nlm.nih.gov/pubmed/20171409.

⑤ Brain Reboot: Harness the Power of Brain Hormones to Transform Your Life

96 **"Often called the 'pleasure chemical,'":** Ed Yong, "The Two Faces of Depression—Two Studies Switch Off Symptoms in Mice But in Opposite Ways," Discover, December 12, 2012. http://blogs.discovermagazine.com/notrocketscience/2012/12/12/the-two-faces-of-depression-two-studies-switch-off-symptoms-in-mice-but-in-opposite-ways/#.XD5sfMHPxPa.

96 **"Things that cause an increase":** "What is Dopamine—And Is It to Blame for Our Addictions?" IFL Science. https://www.iflscience.com/health-and-medicine/what-dopamine-and-it-blame-our-addictions/.

96 **"Dopamine works with serotonin":** Ed Yong, "The Two Faces of Depression—Two Studies Switch Off Symptoms in Mice But in Opposite Ways," Discover, December 12, 2012. http://blogs.discovermagazine.com/notrocketscience/2012/12/12/the-two-faces-of-depression-two-studies-switch-off-symptoms-in-mice-but-in-opposite-ways/#.XD5sfMHPxPa.

96 **"Some of the most common conditions":** Bethany Cadman, "Dopamine deficiency: what you need to know," Medical News Today, January 17, 2018. https://www.medicalnewstoday.com/articles/320637.php.

96 **"Do You Have Low Dopamine Levels?":** Natasha Turner, ND, *The Hormone Diet: A 3-Step Program to Help You Lose Weight, Gain Strength, and Live Younger Longer.* New York: Rodale, 2010, 41. Bethany Cadman, "Dopamine deficiency: what you need to know," Medical News Today, January 17, 2018. https://www.medicalnewstoday.com/articles/320637.php.

97 **"In this study the researchers":** X. N. Lv et al., "Aromatherapy and the central nervous system (CNS): therapeutic mechanism and its associated genes," *Current Drug Targets* 14, no.8 (July 2013): 872–79. https://www.ncbi.nlm.nih.gov/pubmed/23531112.

97 **"It may even hold promise":** M. S. Choi et al., "Essential oils from the medicinal herbs upregulate dopamine transporter in rat pheochromocytoma cells," *Journal of Medicinal Food* 18, no. 10 (October 2015): 1112–20. https://www.ncbi.nlm.nih.gov/pubmed/26295793.

97 **"Research published in the medical journal *Neurology*":** Joshua J. Gagne, PharmD, MS, and Melinda C. Power, BA, "Anti-inflammatory drugs and risk of Parkinson disease" *Neurology* 74, no. 12 (March 23, 2010): 995–1002. https://www.ncbi.nlm.nih.gov/pmc/articles/PMC2848103/.

97 **"But there may be other reasons":** H. Kabuto et al., "Zingerone [4-(4-hydroxy-3-methoxyphenyl)-2-butanone] prevents 6-hydroxydopamine-induced dopamine depression in mouse striatum and increases superoxide scavenging activity in serum," *Neurochemical Research* 30, no. 3 (March 2005): 325–32. https://www.ncbi.nlm.nih.gov/pubmed/16018576.

99 **"A study published in the medical journal *Fundamental and Clinical Pharmacology*":** F. H. Melo et al., "Antidepressant-like effect of carvacrol (5-isopropyl-2 methylphenol) in mice: involvement of dopaminergic system," *Fundamental & Clinical Pharmacology* 25, no. 3 (June 2011): 362–7. https://www.ncbi.nlm.nih.gov/pubmed/20608992.

99 **"Another study found that ingestion":** A. O. Mechan et al., "Monoamine reuptake inhibition and mood-enhancing potential of a specified oregano extract," *British Journal of Nutrition* 105, no. 8 (April 2011): 1150–63. https://www.ncbi.nlm.nih.gov/pubmed/21205415.

99 **"Preliminary animal research published in the medical journal *Phytomedicine*":** N. Zhang et al., "The anxiolytic effect of essential oil of Cananga odorata on exposure of mice and determination of its major active constituents," *Phytomedicine* 23, no. 14 (December 15, 2016): 1727–34. https://www.sciencedirect.com/science/article/pii/S0944711316301908?via%3Dihub.

100 **"Low serotonin levels":** Emily Deans, MD, "Sunlight, Sugar, and Serotonin," https://www.psychologytoday.com/us/blog/evolutionary-psychiatry/201105/sunlight-sugar-and-serotonin; Emil F. Coccaro et al., "Serotonin and impulsive aggression," *CNS Spectrums* 20 (2015): 295–302. Cambridge University Press 2015. doi: 10.1017/S1092852915000310.https://pdfs.semanticscholar.org/481c/3fd12ef726bddba7e5672308c82ef630f10a.pdf.

100 **"Serotonin is involved in":** "3 Types of Muscle Tissue: The Function of Skeletal, Cardiac, and Smooth Muscle," Visible Body. https://www.visiblebody.com/learn/muscular/muscle-types.

100 **"It also helps regulate":** James McIntosh, "What Is Serotonin and What Does It Do?" MedicalNewsToday, August 4, 2011. https://www.medicalnewstoday.com/kc/serotonin-facts-232248.

100 **"Serotonin even helps to reduce":** James McIntosh, "What Is Serotonin and What Does It Do?" MedicalNewsToday, August 4, 2011. https://www.medicalnewstoday.com/kc/serotonin-facts-232248.

100 **"Do You Have Low Serotonin?":** Natasha Turner, ND, *The Hormone Diet: A 3-Step Program to Help You Lose Weight, Gain Strength, and Live Younger Longer.* New York: Rodale, 2010, 42.

100 **"Low levels of the hormone serotonin"**: Ana Sandoiu, "Alzheimer's: low serotonin may drive development," MedicalNewsToday, August 15, 2017. https://www.medicalnewstoday.com/articles/318968.php.

101 **"As you learned earlier"**: X. N. Lv et al., "Aromatherapy and the central nervous system (CNS): therapeutic mechanism and its associated genes," *Current Drug Targets* 14, no. 8 (July 2013): 872–79. https://www.ncbi. nlm.nih.gov/pubmed/23531112.

101 **"In another study, researchers found"**: E. Watanabe et al., "Effects of bergamot (Citrus bergamia (Risso) Wright & Arn.) essential oil aromatherapy on mood states, parasympathetic nervous system activity, and salivary cortisol levels in 41 healthy females," *Forsch Komplementmed* 22, no. 1 (2015): 43–49. https://www.ncbi.nlm.nih.gov/pubmed/25824404.

101 **"This could explain its ability"**: "Lavender oil and serotonin," Doterra. https://www.doterra.com/US/en/blog/science-wellness-lavender-oil-serotonin.

102 **"Research even found that lavender essential oil"**: M. Nikfarjam et al., "The effects of *Lavandula angustifolia* mill infusion on depression in patients using Citalopram: a comparison study," *Iranian Red Crescent Medical Journal* 15, no. 8 (August 2013): 734–39. https://www.ncbi.nlm. nih.gov/pubmed/24578844.

102 **"It also helps to"**: V. Lopez et al., "Exploring pharmacological mechanisms of lavender (*Lavandula angustifolia*) essential oil on central nervous system targets," *Frontiers in Pharmacology* 8 (May 19, 2017): 280. https://www.ncbi.nlm.nih.gov/pubmed/28579958.

102 **"The preliminary study"**: D. Medhat et al., "Evaluation of urinary 8-hydroxy-2-deoxyguanosine level in experimental Alzheimer's disease: impact of carvacrol nanoparticles," *Molecular Biology Reports* 46, no. 4 (August 2019): 4517–27. https://www.ncbi.nlm.nih.gov/pubmed/31209743.

102 **"Wild oregano, *origanum vulgare*"**: Aaron Williams, "Terpene Profile: Carvacrol," MONQ. https://monq.com/eo/terpenes/carvacrol/.

102 **"In a study published in the *Journal of Ethnopharmacology*"**: Nan Zhang et al., "*Cananga odorata* essential oil reverses the anxiety induced by 1-(3-chlorophenyl) piperazine through regulating the MAPK pathway and serotonin system in mice," *Journal of Ethnopharmacology* 219 (June 12, 2018): 23–30. https://www.sciencedirect.com/science/article/pii/S0378874117303483?via%3Dihub.

104 **"Copaiba's high concentration"**: doTERRA Essential Oils, "Dr. Hill Discusses Copaiba and Cannabinoid Benefits." https://www.youtube. com/watch?v=axmJurEhptY&list=PLp3VbOdUkkm3j-E47KpJ_ t9vnwqqcvubB&index=9&fbclid=IwAR3zYaAMMUuxKFbm 29lbht3U8LUwoG7kipXiz8OtXZX1i0op4bSPK0a0Qnc.

104 **"A preliminary study published in the medical journal *Biomedicine & Pharmacotherapy*"**: G. Wang. β-Caryophyllene (BCP) ameliorates MPP+ induced cytotoxicity," *Biomedicine & Pharmacotherapy* 103 (July 2018): 1086–91. https://www.ncbi.nlm.nih.gov/pubmed/?term=B-Caryophyllen e+(BCP)+ameliorates+MPP%2B+induced+cytotoxicity.

104 **"A deficiency of acetylcholine"**: Leslie Taylor, "Copaiba," The Healing Power of Rainforest Plants. http://www.rain-tree.com/copaiba.htm.

104 **"As we learned earlier, brain inflammation"**: A. S. Sayed et al., "Role of 3-Acetyl-11-Keto-Beta-Boswellic acid in counteracting LPS-induced neuroinflammation via modulation of miRNA-155," *Molecular Neurobiology* 55, no. 7 (July 2018): 5798–5808. https://www.ncbi.nlm. nih.gov/pubmed/29079998.

105 **"While the research is still"**: O. Cioanca et al., "Anti-acetylcholinesterase and antioxidant activities of inhaled juniper oil on amyloid beta (1–42)-induced oxidative stress in the rat hippocampus," *Neurochemical Research* 40, no. 5 (May 2015): 952–60. https://www.ncbi.nlm.nih.gov/pubmed/25743585.

105 **"This long-time reputation"**: M. Ozarowski et al., "*Rosmarinus officinalis* L. leaf extract improves memory impairment and affects acetylcholinesterase and butyrylcholinesterase activities in rat brain," *Fitoterapia* 91 (December 2013): 261–71. https://www.ncbi.nlm.nih.gov/pubmed/24080468.

105 **"Rosemary has also been found"**: The George Mateljan Foundation, "Rosemary," The World's Healthiest Foods. http://www.whfoods.com/genpage.php?tname=foodspice&dbid=75.

105 **"Since this brain messenger"**: Peter Houghton, "Activity and Constituents of Sage Relevant to the Potential Treatment of Symptoms of Alzheimer's Disease," *Herbalgram: The Journal of the American Botanical Council* 61 (2004): 38–53. http://cms.herbalgram.org/herbalgram/issue61/article2643. html?ts=1574517175&signature=612de687695af1e4a84d53369672a30 2&ts=1574517176&signature=46d1de70aa49641eb04755c355b37f05.

105 **"In a study published in the *Journal of Ethnopharmacology*"**: Namyata Pathak-Gandhi and Ashok D. B. Vaidya, "Management of Parkinson's Disease in Ayurveda: Medicinal plants and adjuvant measures," *Journal of Ethnopharmacology* 197, no. 2 (February 2, 2017): 46–51. https://www.sciencedirect.com/science/article/pii/S0378874116305463?via%3Dihub.

107 **"A study published in the medical journal *Current Drug Targets*"**: X. N. Lv et al., "Aromatherapy and the central nervous system (CNS): therapeutic mechanism and its associated genes," *Current Drug Targets* 14, no. 8 (July 2013): 872–79. https://www.ncbi.nlm.nih.gov/pubmed/23531112.

107 **"The essential oil most known"**: G. H. Seol et al, "Antidepressant-like effect of *Salvia sclarea* is explained by modulation of dopamine activities in rats," *Journal of Ethnopharmacology* 130, no. 1 (July 6, 2010): 187–90. https://www.ncbi.nlm.nih.gov/pubmed/20441789.

107 **"In another study of menopausal women"**: K. B. Lee et al., "Changes in 5-hydroxytryptamine and cortisol plasma levels in menopausal women after inhalation of clary sage oil," *Phytotherapy Research* 28, no. 11 (November 2014): 1599–1605. https://www.ncbi.nlm.nih.gov/pubmed/24802524.

108 **"In a study published in the *Journal of Psychopharmacology*"**: A. Moussaieff et al., "Incensole acetate reduces depressive-like behavior and modulates hippocampal BDNF and CRF expression of submissive animals," *Journal of Psychopharmacology* 26, no. 12 (December 2012): 1584–93. https://www.ncbi.nlm.nih.gov/pubmed/23015543.

108 **"The study found that lavender"**: M. Nikfarjam et al., "The effects of *Lavandula angustifolia* Mill infusion on depression in patients using citalopram: a comparison study," *Iranian Red Crescent Medical Journal* 15, no. 8 (August 2013): 734–39. https://www.ncbi.nlm.nih.gov/pubmed/24578844.

108 **"Another study found that inhaling"**: M. Kianpour et al., "Effect of lavender scent inhalation on prevention of stress, anxiety, and depression in the postpartum period," *Iranian Journal of Nursing and Midwifery Research* 21, no. 2 (March–April 2016): 197–201. https://www.ncbi.nlm.nih.gov/pubmed/27095995.

108 **"According to a study in the journal *Behavioural Brain Research*"**: M. Komiya et al., "Lemon oil vapor causes an anti-stress effect via modulating the 5-HT and DA activities in mice," *Behavioural Brain Research* 172, no. 2 (September 25, 2006): 240–49. https://www.ncbi.nlm.nih.gov/pubmed/16780969.

108 **"People were evaluated"**: J. Lehrner et al., "Ambient odor of orange in a dental office reduces anxiety and improves mood in female patients," *Physiology & Behavior* 71, no. 1–2 (October 1–15, 2000): 83–86. https://www.ncbi.nlm.nih.gov/pubmed/11134689.

108 **"In the study, published in the *Journal of Ethnopharmacology*"**: D. G. Machado et al., "*Rosmarinus officinalis L.* hydroalcoholic extract, similar to fluoxetine, reverses depressive-like behavior without altering learning deficit in olfactory bulbectomized mice," *Journal of Ethnopharmacology* 143, no. 1 (August 30, 2012): 158–69. https://www.ncbi.nlm.nih.gov/pubmed/22721880.

111 **"One study showed that bergamot"**: E. Watanabe et al., "Effects of bergamot (Citrus bergamia (Risso) Wright & Arn.) essential oil aromatherapy on mood states, parasympathetic nervous system activity, and salivary cortisol levels in 41 healthy females," *Forsch Komplementmed* 22, no. 1 (2015): 43–49. https://www.ncbi.nlm.nih.gov/pubmed/25824404.

111 **"In a study published in the *Journal of Ethnopharmacology*"**: L. R. Chioca et al., "Anxiolytic-like effect of lavender essential oil inhalation in mice: participation of serotonergic but not GABAA/benzodiazepine neurotransmission," *Journal of Ethnopharmacology* 147, no. 2 (May 20, 2013): 412–18. https://www.ncbi.nlm.nih.gov/pubmed/23524167.

111 **"Compare that to diazepam"**: "Diazepam," WebMD. https://www.webmd.com/drugs/2/drug-6306/diazepam-oral/details#side-effects.

111 **"In a study published in the journal *Pharmacology, Biochemistry, & Behavior*"**: T. Umezu, "Anti-conflict effects of plant-derived essential oils," *Pharmacology, Biochemistry, & Behavior* 64, no. 1 (September 1999): 35–40. https://www.ncbi.nlm.nih.gov/pubmed/10494995.

111 **"Inhalation of vetiver essential oil"**: S. Sayudthong et al. "Anxiety-like behaviour and c-fos expression in rats that inhaled vetiver essential oil," *Natural Product Research* 29, no. 22 (2015): 2141–44. https://www.ncbi.nlm.nih.gov/pubmed/25553641.

116 **"Here are some of the many health benefits"**: Environmental Health Network, "Twenty Most Common Chemicals Found in Thirty-One Fragrance Products," Environmental Health Network. http://ehnca.org/www/ehn20.htm.

6 Ovary Renewal: The Hormones of Womanhood

123 **"To alleviate mood-related PMS"**: T. Matsumoto et al., "Does lavender aromatherapy alleviate premenstrual emotional symptoms?: a randomized crossover trial" *BioPsychoSocial Medicine* 31, no. 7 (May 31, 2013): 12. http://www.ncbi.nlm.nih.gov/pubmed/23724853.

123 **"In an animal study published in the *Journal of Ethnopharmacology*"**: S. N. Ostad et al., "The effect of fennel essential oil on uterine contraction as a model for dysmenorrhea, pharmacology and toxicology study," *Journal of Ethnopharmacology* 76, no. 3 (August 2001): 299–304. https://www.ncbi.nlm.nih.gov/pubmed/11448553.

123 **"Another study published in the *Iranian Journal of Nursing and Midwifery Research*"**: Masoomeh Nasehi et al., "Comparison of the effectiveness of combination of fennel extract/vitamin E with ibuprofen on the pain intensity in students with primary dysmenorrhea" *Iranian Journal of Nursing and Midwifery Research* 18, no. 5 (September/October 2013): 355–59. https://www.ncbi.nlm.nih.gov/pmc/articles/PMC3877456/.

128 **"Lavender essential oil has been found"**: P. Sasannejad et al., "Lavender essential oil in the treatment of migraine headache: a placebo-controlled clinical trial," *European Neurology* 67, no. 5 (2012): 288–291. https://www.karger.com/Article/Abstract/335249.

128 **"Research in the medical journal *Complementary Therapies in Medicine*"**: M. Niazi et al., "Efficacy of topical rose (Rosa damascene Mill.) oil for migraine headache: A randomized, double-blinded, placebo-controlled cross-over trial," *Complementary Therapies in Medicine*, 34 (October 2017): 35–41. https://www.ncbi.nlm.nih.gov/pubmed/28917373.

130 **"She collected evidence"**: Ethel Burns, et al., "An investigation into the use of aromatherapy in intrapartum midwifery practice," *Journal of Alternative and Complementary Medicine* 6, no. 2 (2000): 141–47.

131 **"According to research published in the *Journal of Caring Sciences*"**: A. Ghiasi et al., "A systematic review on the anxiolytic effect of aromatherapy during the first stage of labor," *Journal of Caring Sciences* 8, no. 1 (March 1, 2019): 51-60. https://www.ncbi.nlm.nih.gov/pubmed/30915314.

132 **"In a study published in the journal *Neuroendocrinology Letters*"**: K. Shinohara et al., "Effects of essential oil exposure on salivary estrogen concentration in perimenopausal women," *Neuroendocrinology Letters* 37, no. 8 (January 2017): 567–72. https://www.ncbi.nlm.nih.gov/pubmed/28326753.

134 **"In a study published in the journal *Neuroendocrinology Letters*"**: K. Shinohara et al., "Effects of essential oil exposure on salivary estrogen concentration in perimenopausal women," *Neuroendocrinology Letters* 37, no. 8 (January 2017): 567–72. https://www.ncbi.nlm.nih.gov/pubmed/28326753.

135 **"Stick with it"**: V. Farnia et al., "Adjuvant Rosa Damascena has a small effect on SSSI-induced sexual dysfunction in female patients suffering from MDD," *Pharmacopsychiatry* 48, no. 4–5 (July 2015): 156–63. https://www.ncbi.nlm.nih.gov/pubmed/26098128.

137 **"Do You Have Low Estrogen Levels?"**: Natasha Turner, *The Hormone Diet: A 3-Step Program to Help You Lose Weight, Gain Strength, and Live Younger Longer.* New York: Rodale, 2010, 46.

137 **"Postpartum depression"**: "Estrogen and Women's Emotions," WebMD. https://www.webmd.com/women/guide/estrogen-and-womens-emotions#2.

141 **"Estrogen dominance can be linked":** Jayne Leonard, "What are the symptoms of high estrogen?" WebMD. https://www.medicalnewstoday.com/articles/323280.php.

141 **"Their symptoms typically include":** Jayne Leonard, "What are the symptoms of high estrogen?" WebMD. https://www.medicalnewstoday.com/articles/323280.php.

143 **"This delightfully smelling essential oil":** *The Essential Life: 3rd Edition.* Total Wellness Publishing, LLC: 2017, 304.

143 **"It is also a good essential oil":** *The Essential Life: 3rd Edition.* Total Wellness Publishing, LLC: 2017, 304.

143 **"Best known for its antiviral":** D. T. Dava et al., "Estrogen and progestin bioactivity of foods, herbs, and spices," *Proceedings of the Society for Experimental Biology and Medicine* 369, no. 3 (March 1998): 369–78. https://www.ncbi.nlm.nih.gov/pubmed/9492350.

143 **"Like oregano, thyme is a powerful":** D. T. Dava et al., "Estrogen and progestin bioactivity of foods, herbs, and spices," *Proceedings of the Society for Experimental Biology and Medicine* 217, no. 3 (March 1998): 369–78. https://www.ncbi.nlm.nih.gov/pubmed/9492350.

143 **"This brilliant yellow Indian essential oil":** D. T. Dava et al., "Estrogen and progestin bioactivity of foods, herbs, and spices," *Proceedings of the Society for Experimental Biology and Medicine* 217, no. 3 (March 1998): 369–78. https://www.ncbi.nlm.nih.gov/pubmed/9492350.

144 **"Research in the journal *Fertility and Sterility*":** H. Henmi et al., "Effects of ascorbic acid supplementation on serum progesterone levels in patients with a luteal phase defect," *Fertility and Sterility* 80, no. 2 (August 2003): 459–61. https://www.ncbi.nlm.nih.gov/pubmed/12909517.

145 **"In a study of women with low progesterone":** L. M. Westphal et al., "Double-blind, placebo-controlled study of Fertilityblend: a nutritional supplement for improving fertility in women," *Clinical and Experimental Obstetrics and Gynecology* 33, no. 4 (2006): 205–8. https://www.ncbi.nlm.nih.gov/pubmed/17211965.

145 **"Some of the best foods":** Rachel Nall, "How to Naturally Increase Your Progesterone Levels," Healthline. https://www.healthline.com/health/natural-progesterone.

146 **"While there isn't a lot of research":** Sadeghi Altaabadi M. et al., "Role of essential oil *Mentha spicata* (spearmint) in addressing reverse hormonal and folliculogenesis disturbances in a polycystic ovarian syndrome in a rat model." *Advanced Pharmaceutical Bulletin* 7, no. 4 (December 2017): 651–54. https://www.ncbi.nlm.nih.gov/pubmed/29399556.

147 **"Geranium essential oil contains esters":** Kurt Schnaubelt, *Advanced Aromatherapy: The Science of Essential Oil Therapy*, Rochester, Vermont: Healing Arts Press, 1998, 70.

147 **"According to the *Indian Journal of Dentistry*":** H. Rahman and A. Chandra, "Microbiologic evaluation of *matricaria* and chlorhexidine against *E. faecalis* and *C. albicans*," *Indian Journal of Dentistry* 6, no. 2 (April–June 2015): 60–64. https://www.ncbi.nlm.nih.gov/pubmed/26097333.

147 **"A well-established antifungal herb":** M. S. Khan et al., "Sub-MICs of *Carum copticum* and *Thymus vulgaris* influence virulence factors and biofilm formation in *Candida spp.*," *BMC Complementary and Alternative Medicine* 14 (September 15, 2014): 337. https://www.ncbi.nlm.nih.gov/pubmed/25220750.

 7 **The Male Rebuild:**
The DIY Hormone Solution for Men's Vigor and Vitality

150 **"There are many signs":** Ryan Wallace and Kathleen Yoder, "12 Signs of Low Testosterone," Healthline. https://www.healthline.com/health/low-testosterone/warning-signs.

150 **"Erectile dysfunction (on its own)":** Ryan Wallace and Kathleen Yoder, "12 Signs of Low Testosterone," Healthline. https://www.healthline.com/health/low-testosterone/warning-signs#erections.

151 **"Research shows that regular ingestion":** Al-Kadir Mares et al., "The effect of ginger on semen parameters and serum FSH, LH and testosterone of infertile men," *Tikrit Medical Journal* 18, no. 2 (December 2012): 322. http://connection.ebscohost.com/c/articles/98039248/effect-ginger-semen-parameters-serum-fsh-lh-testosterone-infertile-men.

153 **"As a result, it's far more common":** Charles Patrick Davis, "High and low testosterone levels in men," MedicineNet. https://www.medicinenet.com/high_and_low_testosterone_levels_in_men/views.htm.

154 **"While the study assessed the oil's effect":** Sadeghi Altaabadi M. et al., "Role of essential oil *Mentha spicata* (spearmint) in addressing reverse hormonal and folliculogenesis disturbances in a polycystic ovarian syndrome in a rat model," *Advanced Pharmaceutical Bulletin* 7, no. 4 (December 2017): 651–54. https://www.ncbi.nlm.nih.gov/pubmed/29399556.

155 **"In a study published in the *European Journal of Applied Physiology*":** D. Vaamonde et al., "Physically active men show better sperm parameters and hormone values than sedentary men," *European Journal of Applied Physiology* 112, no. 9 (September 2012): 3267–73. https://www.ncbi.nlm.nih.gov/pubmed/22234399.

155 **"Another study published in the *Journal of Clinical Biochemistry and Nutrition*":** H. Kumagai et al., "Increased physical activity has a greater effect than reduced energy intake on lifestyle-modification induced increases in testosterone," *Journal of Clinical Biochemistry and Nutrition* 58, no. 1 (January 2016): 84–89. https://www.ncbi.nlm.nih.gov/pubmed/26798202.

155 **"According to research in the *Journal of Ayub Medical College*":** G. M. Lodhi et al., "Effects of ascorbic acid and alpha tocopherol supplementation on acute restraint stress-induced changes in testosterone, corticosterone, and norepinephrine levels in male Sprague Dawley rats," *Journal of Ayub Medical College* 26, no. 1 (January–March 2015): 7–11. https://www.ncbi.nlm.nih.gov/pubmed/25358206.

155 **"Published in the *Journal of the American Medical Association*":** R. Leproult and E. Van Cauter. "Effect of one week of sleep restriction on testosterone levels in young, healthy men," *JAMA* 305, no. 21 (June 1, 2011): 2173–74. https://www.ncbi.nlm.nih.gov/pubmed/21632481.

155 **"In a year-long study":** S. Pilz et al., "Effect of vitamin D supplementation on testosterone levels in men," *Hormone and Metabolic Research* 43, no. 3 (March 2011): 223–35. https://www.ncbi.nlm.nih.gov/pubmed/21154195.

156 **"In a study published in *Renal Failure*":** G. R. Jalali et al., "Impact of oral zinc therapy on the level of sex hormones in male patients on hemodialysis," *Renal Failure* 32, no. 4 (May 2010): 417–19. https://www.ncbi.nlm.nih.gov/pubmed/20446777.

156 **"Another study published in the *Journal of Human Reproductive Sciences*":** D. M. A. B. Dissanayake et al., "Effects of zinc supplementation on sexual behavior of male rats," *Journal of Human Reproductive Sciences* 2, no.2 (July–December 2009): 57–61. https://www.ncbi.nlm.nih.gov/pmc/articles/PMC2800928/.

156 **"In a study published in *Fertility and Sterility*":** W. Y. Wong et al., "Effects of folic acid and zinc sulfate on male factor subfertility: a double-blind, randomized, placebo-controlled trial," *Fertility and Sterility* 77, no. 3 (March 2001): 491–18. https://www.ncbi.nlm.nih.gov/pubmed/11872201.

156 **"A study published in the *International Journal of Fertility & Sterility*":** B. Rahmati et al,. "Effect of *Withania somnifera (L.) Dunal* on sex hormone and gonadotropin levels in addicted male rats," *International Journal of Fertility & Sterility* 10, no. 2 (July–September, 2016): 239–44. https://www.ncbi.nlm.nih.gov/pubmed/27441058.

157 **"Compounds found in frankincense":** H. Q. Yuan et al., "Inhibitory effect of acetyl-11-keto-beta-boswellic acid on androgen receptor by interference of Sp1 binding activity in prostate cancer cells," *Biochemical Pharmacology* 75, no. 11 (June 1, 2008): 2112–21. https://www.ncbi.nlm.nih.gov/pubmed/18430409.

157 **"Juniper essential oil is best known":** *The Essential Life: 3rd Edition.* Total Wellness Publishing: 2017, 277.

157 **"A study published in the *Journal of Food Biochemistry*":** A. M. El-Wakf et al, "Marjoram and sage oils protect against testicular apoptosis, suppressed Ki-67 expression and cell cycle arrest as a therapy for male infertility in the obese rats," *Journal of Food Biochemistry*, 44, no. 1 (January 2020). https://www.ncbi.nlm.nih.gov/pubmed/31612531.

157 **"According to research in the *International Journal of Fertility & Sterility*":** M. Soltani et al., "Protective effects of *Matricaria chamomilla* extract on torsion/detorsion-induced tissue damage and oxidative stress in adult rat testes," *International Journal of Fertility & Sterility* 12, no. 3 (June 2018): 242–48. https://www.ncbi.nlm.nih.gov/pubmed/29935071.

157 **"According to research in the *Journal of Dietary Supplements*":** S. Hamedi et al, "Rosa damascena Mill. Essential oil has protective effect against testicular damage in diabetic rats," *Journal of Dietary Supplements* 15, no. 3 (May 4, 2018): 311–17. https://www.ncbi.nlm.nih.gov/pubmed/28792252.

157 **Research in the journal *Phytomedicine*":** A. J. Bommareddy et al., "α-santalol, a derivative of sandalwood oil, induces apoptosis in human prostate cancer cells by causing caspase-3 activation," *Phytomedicine* 19, no. 8–9 (June 15, 2012): 804–11. https://www.sciencedirect.com/science/article/abs/pii/S0944711312001250?via%3Dihub.

158 **"In a study published in the journal *Food Science & Nutrition*":** S. Perna et al., "Efficacy of bergamot: From anti-inflammatory and anti-oxidative mechanisms to clinical applications as preventive agent for cardiovascular morbidity, skin diseases, and mood alterations," *Food Science & Nutrition* 7, no. 2 (January 25, 2019): 369–84. https://www.ncbi.nlm.nih.gov/pubmed/30847114.

158 **"Research published in the *International Journal of Pharmaceutical Sciences and Research*":** R. Kaushik, D. Gupta, and R. Yadav, "Alopecia: Herbal Remedies," *International Journal of Pharmaceutical Sciences and Research*, May 21, 2011. https://www.researchgate.net/profile/Rahul_Kaushik4/publication/215800523_ALOPECIA_HERBAL_REMEDIES/links/02865134e9e0c1ab0b484751.pdf.

158 **"Scientists found that the rosemary extract":** K. Murata et al., "Promotion of hair growth by Rosmarinus officinalis leaf extract," *Phytotherapy Research* 27, no. 2 (February 2013): 212–17. https://www.ncbi.nlm.nih.gov/pubmed/22517595.

160 **"Research shows that regular ingestion":** Al-Kadir Mares et al., "The effect of ginger on semen parameters and serum FSH, LH, & testosterone of infertile men," *Tikrit Medical Journal* 18, no. 2 (2012): 322. http://connection.ebscohost.com/c/articles/98039248/effect-ginger-semen-parameters-serum-fsh-lh-testosterone-infertile-men.

160 **"Research shows that regular inhalation":** E. Kose et al., "Rose oil inhalation protects against formaldehyde-induced testicular damage in rats," *Andrologia* 44, Suppl 1 (May 2012): 342–48. https://www.ncbi.nlm.nih.gov/pubmed/21749434.

160 **"Because rose can protect":** M. Askaripour et al., "The effect of aqueous extract of *Rosa damascena* on formaldehyde-induced toxicity in mice testes," *Pharmaceutical Biology* 56, no. 1 (December 2018): 12–17. https://www.ncbi.nlm.nih.gov/pubmed/29231061.

161 **"A study published in the *Journal of Cellular Biochemistry*":** A. P. Ames-Sibin et al., "β-caryophyllene, the major constituent of copaiba oil, reduces systemic inflammation and oxidative stress in arthritic rats," *Journal of Cellular Biochemistry* 119, no. 2 (December 2018): 10262–77. https://www.ncbi.nlm.nih.gov/pubmed/30132972.

161 **"A study published in the *Journal of the American Mosquito Control Association*":** R. M. Castillo et al., "Insecticidal and repellent activity of several plant-derived essential oils against aedes aegypti," *Journal of the American Mosquito Control Association* 33, no. 1 (March 2017): 25–35. https://www.ncbi.nlm.nih.gov/pubmed/28388322.

162 **"A study published in *Natural Products Research*":** J. F. Carroll et al., "Repellency of the *Origanum onites L.* essential oil and constituents to the lone star tick and yellow fever mosquito," *Natural Products Research* 31, no. 18 (September 2017): 2192–97. https://www.ncbi.nlm.nih.gov/pubmed/28278656.

162 **"Compare that to the findings":** Susan Brink, "What's the Best Way to Keep Mosquitoes from Biting?" NPR, January 30, 2016. https://www.npr.org/sections/goatsandsoda/2016/01/30/464740275/whats-the-best-way-to-keep-mosquitoes-from-biting.

Essential Oil Usage Chart

164 *The Essential Life: 3rd Edition.* Total Wellness Publishing, LLC: 2017.

PICTURE CREDITS

INDEX

NOTE: Page numbers in *italics* indicate/include recipes. Page numbers in parentheses indicate noncontiguous references.

ABOUT THE AUTHOR

Michelle Schoffro Cook, PhD, DNM, RNCP, is an international best-selling and 24-time book author whose works include *The Essential Oils Healing Deck*, *Be Your Own Herbalist*, *60 Seconds to Slim*, *The Ultimate pH Solution*, and *The Cultured Cook*. She is a board-certified doctor of natural medicine, registered nutritionist, certified herbalist, and aromatherapist. Her books are distributed worldwide and have been translated into many languages, including Greek, Chinese, Indonesian, Russian, Spanish, Thai, and others.

Her blogs and articles have been featured in or on Care2.com, Yahoo!, *Mother Earth Living*, *Fermentation*, Huffington Post, and *alive* magazine. Dr. Cook's work has appeared in *Woman's World* magazine, *First for Women* magazine, WebMD, Reviews.com, *Closer Weekly*, *The Vancouver Sun*, Thrive Global, *Hello!* magazine, *Vegetarian Times*, *Glow*, the *Ottawa Citizen*, the *Calgary Herald*, and many other publications and sites.

She is the publisher of the popular free health e-newsletter *World's Healthiest News* that reaches over 10,000 readers in over 100 countries worldwide. Discover how to maximize the healing power of essential oils by joining Dr. Cook's Medical Aromatherapy team, available through her website at DrMichelleCook.com/JoinMyTeam.

Learn more about Dr. Cook's work at: DrMichelleCook.com, FoodHouseProject.com, and LostOrchard.org.

Connect with Dr. Cook at: Instagram (@DrMichelleCook), Facebook (DrMichelleCook and DrSchoffroCook), and Twitter (@mschoffrocook).